Springer Series on
# REHABILITATION

Editor: Thomas E. Backer, Ph.D.
Human Interaction Research Institute, Los Angeles

Advisory Board:

Carolyn L. Vash, Ph.D., Elizabeth L. Pan, Ph.D., Donald E. Galvin, Ph.D.,
Ray L. Jones, Ph.D., James F. Garrett, Ph.D., Patricia G. Forsythe,
and Henry Viscardi, Jr.

**Elaine Greif** completed her B.A. in Philosophy and Psychology at the University of Rochester and her M.A. and Ph.D. in Clinical Psychology at Arizona State University. She completed her clinical internship at the Medical School, Oregon Health Sciences University. Since 1978, she has been a member of the Department of Health Care Psychology at Emanuel Hospital in Portland, Oregon. Her primary interests are clinical neuropsychology and the application of psychological principles in medical and rehabilitation settings. At the Emanuel Rehabilitation Center, she is particularly active in work with adults who have suffered traumatic brain injuries.

**Ruth G. Matarazzo** received her B.A. from Brown University and her M.A. and Ph.D. from Washington University (St. Louis) in Clinical Psychology. Subsequently, she held research fellowships at Washington University School of Medicine and Harvard Medical School and has been on the faculty at the Medical School, Oregon Health Sciences University since 1957, where she is currently Professor of Medical Psychology. She is a Fellow of A.P.A., an A.B.P.P. diplomate, and has held offices in local, regional, and national psychological associations. Her interests and her research have included teaching of interviewing skills, neuropsychology, and other aspects of clinical psychology as applied to medical settings.

# Behavioral Approaches to Rehabilitation

## Coping with Change

**Elaine Greif, Ph.D.**
**Ruth G. Matarazzo, Ph.D.**

Foreword by Lee Meyerson, Ph.D.

**Springer Publishing Company**
**New York**

Springer Publishing Company, Inc.
200 Park Avenue South
New York, New York 10003

82 83 84 85 86/ 10 9 8 7 6 5 4 3 2 1

---

**Library of Congress Cataloging in Publication Data**

Greif, Elaine.
  Behavioral approaches to rehabilitation.

  (Springer series on rehabilitation; v. 3)
  Bibliography: p.
  Includes index.
    1. Rehabilitation.   2. Handicapped—Psychology.
I. Matarazzo, Ruth G.   II. Title.   III. Series.
[DNLM: 1. Behavior.   2. Chronic disease—Psychology.
3. Chronic disease—Rehabilitation.   4. Rehabilita-
tion—Psychology.   5. Handicapped—Psychology.
W1 SP685SF v. 3 / WB 320 G824b]
RM930.G74          617          81-16689
ISBN 0-8261-3530-7          AACR2
ISBN 0-8261-3531-5 (pbk.)

---

Printed in the United States of America

# CONTENTS

# FOREWORD

Rehabilitation is a relatively new field of treatment, specialization, and investigation. Even more recent is the systematic application of this increasing knowledge generated by experience and experiment.

Gradually, the experimental data, the experienced professional wisdom, and the several philosophical approaches relating to helping human beings who have experienced physical and psychological damage—which previously were known only to readers of the technical journal literature in rehabilitation—are being organized into book-length expositions.

There are now several elementary and advanced text and reference books for students and practitioners in the helping professions that transmit knowledge related to rehabilitation to wider audiences. Some books identify and describe what each profession contributes to the complex task of returning ill and disabled people to meaningful and fulfilling lives, some show the kinds of services that are needed in treating each of a multitude of specific organic impairments, and some discuss the meaning and problems of disability in general. Other books examine critically the expanding experimental literature, with its inevitable mixture of congruent and noncongruent results, and try to distinguish conclusions that can be considered reasonably established from plausible but unproved, or flawed, work. An abundance of book-length compilations of selected reprints assists the neophyte in becoming sensitized to the many problems faced by disabled persons and in experiencing vicariously the triumphs and losses of the rehabilitation process. Until now, however, there has been no book that introduces students and professionals to the world of the rehabilitation hospital, explains some of the barriers to successful treatment, and proposes some good solutions in explicit detail.

Drs. Greif and Matarazzo have written a very practical and therapeutically useful book. Here, they say, is an overview of some common patterns of behavior we have found among clients in a rehabilitation setting, these are some of the things a professional can and should do to help, and—uniquely—

*this is how you do it*. They give the reader an effective orientation to social psychological phenomena that rehabilitation workers previously had to learn by trial and error on the job or from the verbal and behavioral modeling of insightful, experienced mentors. Their exposition closely approaches the freeflowing supervisory discourse of an able and experienced rehabilitation professional, and the result is likely to be useful to all who work with patients and their families.

Although their approach is primarily behavioral, the authors are rarely doctrinaire. Those who prefer humanistic, phenomenological, cognitive, or personality-oriented approaches will find some implicit consideration of these views and much that can be restated in nonbehavioral language. The authors make it clear that analysis of behavior and knowledge of the principles of learning are effective tools for aiding patients. They do not require a belief that disability reduces a person to a manipulable cipher. On the contrary, they emphasize that patients are reasonable human beings who make the professional's task easier and more effective if they are treated with respect and allowed reasonable autonomy and control. The behavioral analysis of patient motivation—a central problem in every rehabilitation setting I know—is particularly good.

One limitation of a freewheeling manual of therapeutics arises from the same characteristic that contributes to its readability and interest: It is not cluttered with citations. The format does not permit an immediate response to questions (sometimes challenges) of an alert reader to particular statements or points of view; namely, "Do we really know that? What is the evidence?"

Unlike the researcher, writing for other researchers, who wishes to document every conclusion drawn, the practicing clinician must function with the beliefs and procedures that experience has shown to be useful. The reader must understand, therefore, that although much of what is in this book is based on reasonably rigorous evidence, there are also statements and points of view that may not receive universal assent.

Unquestionably, however, the instructor who delights in showing students the relevant evidence and in stimulating research-oriented discussion will find this an exciting and highly "teachable" book. Health professionals and caretakers who absorb the rationale and follow the therapeutic strategies advocated by Drs. Greif and Matarazzo will find that their improved skills are promptly reflected in the progress of their patients.

Lee Meyerson, Ph.D.
Arizona State University
Tempe, Arizona

# ACKNOWLEDGMENTS

We would like to express our appreciation to friends and colleagues who supported our writing this book. We thank Cindy Buckley, O.T.R., Carole Curran, Irene Greif, Ph.D., Kenneth Kasner, Ph.D., Sue Kingsbury, R.N., May Rawlinson, Ph.D., and Greg Terranova for their comments on our manuscript. We offer special thanks to Laurence Binder, Ph.D. for his extensive comments on the chapter about brain injury.

We also appreciate the excellent secretarial assistance we received from Lyle Earl; Barbara Hicks; Judy Maxey; Cindi Norsworthy and Frances Johnson at Emanuel Hospital; and Molly Sorensen, Lois Holland, and Laurel Palanuk at the University of Oregon Health Sciences Center.

We are particularly grateful to those patients and their families who allowed us to describe their situations in order to assist our readers.

# INTRODUCTION

*Behavioral Approaches to Rehabilitation* is designed to be a practical hand-book for therapists and caretakers of patients whose functioning has been impaired by injury or disease. It should prove useful to those working in acute-care hospitals, rehabilitation settings, extended-care facilities, nursing homes, and patients' private homes. In all of these settings the primary goals of treatment are to help patients regain medical stability and to return, as nearly as possible, to their prior levels of functioning.

Although every disease or injury is associated with its own specific causes, deficits, treatments, and prognosis, there are significant shared elements in the psychological and social ramifications of any catastrophic medical condition. In particular, the chronic nature of disabling conditions contributes to the patients' experiencing many similar personal, familial, and social changes. Due to modern medicine's increasingly effective treatment, there are greater numbers of "survivors" of acute medical crises, people who must confront these changes. For these reasons, we have chosen to focus this book upon the psychosocial aspects of disability that may be common among patients with disparate organic impairments.

There are two basic areas of focus throughout the book: (1) the patterns of behavior that rehabilitation patients (and the people working with such patients) commonly display and (2) the principles of human learning and behavior that caretakers can apply in order to understand and facilitate patients' adjustment.

In Part I, we describe what constitutes rehabilitation (Chapter 1) and discuss general psychological processes that are observed in patients as they respond and adjust to their disabilities (Chapter 2).

In Part II, we present some fundamental principles of behavior and the ways in which, during rehabilitation, environmental conditions can shape behavior to become either more or less adaptive. Thus, Chapter 3 describes the social, interpersonal, and private (feelings and thoughts) events that influence learning and behavior; while Chapter 4 focuses on physical environments and the ways in which they can be designed for the patient's practical advantage and better adjustment.

In Part III, we consider patterns of behavior (or groups of particular kinds of patients) that present special challenges during rehabilitation. We use the behavioral principles, introduced earlier, to begin to understand maladaptive patterns of behavior and to develop therapeutic strategies to ameliorate them and facilitate patients' adjustment. In Chapters 5 through 10, we discuss patients who are depressed, anxious, demanding and complaining, "unmotivated," brain-injured, and disoriented. In these chapters, we present information on brain functioning and the cognitive, emotional, and behavioral consequences of brain dysfunction. Included are behavioral descriptions of patients' neuropsychologic deficits and suggested behavioral approaches for use in shaping adaptive behavior within the limits set by neurologic damage. In the final chapters of this section, we discuss areas of particular concern in the rehabilitation of aged patients (Chapter 11) and of children and young adults (Chapter 12).

In Part IV, we move on to the experiences of caretakers, including patients' families (Chapter 13) and rehabilitation professionals (Chapter 14). We emphasize that these "significant others" must cope personally with a range of stresses associated with rehabilitation and must respond therapeutically to patients' needs. We consider typical stresses experienced by caretakers and, from a behavioral perspective, suggest ways for family members and health professionals both to support optimal adjustment by patients and to cope with their own demanding roles.

Finally, in the Epilogue, we present a detailed case history describing one patient's presenting medical, psychological, and behavioral difficulties and the treatment strategies that were used during rehabilitation. We review the patient's response to treatment and progress in the hospital, at home, and in the community, highlighting both the separate and the interactive roles of the patient, health professionals, family, friends, and community agencies.

In the Appendixes, we offer examples of treatment approaches suggested in the text and some ways to identify appropriate community resources. These include details on methods of charting progress in treatment (Appendix A), effective use of rewards and praise (Appendix B), scheduling a patient's routine (Appendix C), teaching a method of relaxation (Appendix D), and using community resources for information, support, and action (Appendix E).

We expect that our readers will acquire increased understanding of patients' psychological functioning; ideas on how to approach a variety of situations in patient care; and strategies to increase personal effectiveness and satisfaction in working with patients and their families during rehabilitation. We add a cautionary note, however, that those working with seriously impaired patients cannot always expect rapid, heartening results. Despite one's best and competent efforts, it may take months or years, depending upon the extent of the patient's losses and the probability of her return to at least moderate independence, for the patient (and family members) to achieve satisfactory adjustment. Indeed, when a person's deficits are particularly great, a limited return of function may be all that is possible. Physical obstacles as well as negative attitudes and discrimination within the community also can limit the disabled person's complete reintegration into her natural environment. We believe, however, that even these less fortunate outcomes can be accepted when rehabilitation workers gain rewards from many patients' greater successes and from remembering that their team offers its best efforts in all situations.

# I

# Overview of Rehabilitation

# 1    What Rehabilitation Is

Rehabilitation is the learning process by which a person who has suffered physical, intellectual, and/or personality changes (secondary to injury or disease) recovers functioning to the extent possible, develops compensatory skills in areas where deficits persist, and adjusts emotionally to the level of functioning attained. Thus, rehabilitation is concerned with the patient's optimal physical recovery, reestablishment of skills, and achievement of a satisfactory quality of life.

Comprehensive rehabilitation is a multifaceted effort. It involves evaluation of a patient's functioning and often long-term treatment in areas such as mobility, self-care, communication, personal and family adjustment, sexuality, vocational and avocational planning, and social integration. Specific goals in each of these areas are shaped by the needs that are expressed by the patient, those who are intimately involved with him,* as well as by the suggestions from rehabilitation specialists. Professional contributions typically come from physicians (particularly a physiatrist, who is a physician with a specialty in rehabilitation medicine), nurses, psychologists, occupational therapists, physical therapists, speech and language pathologists, social workers, vocational counselors, and recreational therapists.

Although the focus of rehabilitation is primarily on the patient, the family and extended social network (friends, coworkers) also must be considered. As we know, most individuals belong to a social system in which each member's life influences the lives of other members; thus, significant disruptions and, in turn, the need for adjustments, may befall several members of a social system as the result of one member's impairment. In a family, for example, disability suffered by one person typically demands that other family members accommodate the new circumstances and cope with the loved one's misfor-

---

*Throughout this book, we alternate the use of female and male pronouns to avoid the bias implicit in using either gender alone, or the cumbersome result of using them in combination (e.g., himself/herself).

tune. In such a case, the family's positive adjustment becomes a goal during rehabilitation, both as a worthy aim in itself and because it, in turn, can enhance the patient's progress.

## Rehabilitation Strategies

*Reestablishing the Patient's Premorbid Skills.*   The most desirable goal following any impairment, of course, is complete or near complete recovery. In this case, the patient is expected to recover spontaneously or relearn all or almost all previously established skills and to be able to manage in nearly all situations much as he did prior to disability. For example, a return to full pre-morbid functioning, often with minimal rehabilitative efforts, is expected among patients who require only acute medical care, who break a bone, undergo routine surgery, or suffer burns which will heal completely. Patients with more disabling conditions also may regain functioning sufficiently to perform selected activities, although with some decrement in skill. For example, following a stroke, a person may relearn to talk clearly, walk independently, or write with his preferred hand, although these may not be done as steadily, quickly, or gracefully as before.

*Teaching the Patient New Skills for Achieving Previous Goals.*   When a person is unable to re-establish specific skills which have been impaired, alternate, compensatory skills may be identified and developed in the service of attaining previously developed goals. For example, when a patient's neurologic or orthopedic difficulty renders walking impossible, another manner of achieving independent mobility should be targeted: namely, the independent use of a wheelchair. As previously, the patient will be able to get around his apartment and the community, but will need to learn how to do so with a wheelchair. Similarly, if a patient's ability to speak remains impaired after an injury, he can be taught to use non-oral means of communication such as gesturing and writing (see Chapters 4 and 9). Or, if he loses an arm, or it becomes restricted in movement or strength, vocational retraining would be essential in order to enable him to return to competitive employment. In the last two examples, new skills must be developed if the patient is to regain his earlier capabilities to communicate and maintain gainful employment, respectively.

*Setting New Goals and Facilitating Their Achievement.*   When one ability that is essential to perform a task, or several abilities that include all alternate ways to perform that task, are impaired, the patient must be helped to accept the loss of that function and identify new, attainable goals. For example, if physical injury severely limits motor control or coordination, it may not be possible to participate in sports such as jogging, tennis, or skiing. In this case, it would be important for the sports-oriented patient to identify and pursue activities more amenable to motoric limitations, such as fishing or swimming. In addition, the patient might develop new, substitute interests, such as reading, listening to music, collecting stamps, and other less active endeavors. Similarly, when multiple severe deficits render competitive employment impossible, the patient must develop alternate goals that will generate and support meaningful activity, social contacts, and daily structure, all of which were gained previously through work. Toward these goals, it might be planned for the patient to participate in a day-treatment program, a supervised workshop or activities center, or a volunteer organization.

*Facilitating the Patient's Adjustment.*  The patient probably has to face changes in abilities, activities, and roles in the family and community as a result of disabilities. Positive adjustment is accomplished when a person accepts, although she cannot be expected to like, these changes and losses; recognizes her abilities as well as her disabilities, her assets as well as her limitations; and functions in the world at a level commensurate with retained abilities. Assessing whether a person's adjustment is healthy should involve a relatively objective judgment of the extent to which her behavior helps or hinders immediate and long-term prospects for recovery of function and for life satisfaction.

*Facilitating the Family's Adjustment.*  When a person's functioning is impaired, family members often change, at least in part, their relationships, routines, and responsibilities. This requires that the family understand both how the patient has changed and how she is still the same; in which areas she will be limited, and in which areas she will continue to be competent. Due to the patient's limitations, families typically will have to forego some previous sources of satisfaction and assume additional responsibilities. For example, the husband who rarely cooked a meal may need to learn kitchen skills if his wife no longer can practice them. Similarly, children who have depended on their father for transportation may learn to take buses and to accept missing some activities to which they cannot find transportation. In addition, family members may have to care for the patient, witness the loved one's limitations and associated distress, and share the anxiety of an uncertain future. Family adjustment regarding each of these issues must be an integral part of rehabilitation goals (see Chapter 13).

## The Course of Rehabilitation

Rehabilitation begins immediately following the stabilization of an acute medical crisis. The crisis, which results in some loss of functioning, can be associated with an injury, a single medical episode of a nonprogressive disease, or an exacerbation of symptoms during the course of chronic, progressive illness (see Chapter 2). Although rehabilitative efforts usually are most intense and most apparent as a discrete course of treatment during the period immediately following acute care, rehabilitation can be considered "in progress" as long as the disabled person attempts to improve impaired skills and to approach more closely his premorbid level of functioning. Certainly, rehabilitation is not limited to specified treatments with professionals or to activities designed in rehabilitation programs. Rather, these treatments provide only the foundation from which to stimulate and guide the major work of rehabilitation, which occurs in the community, at home, in the workplace, and so on. It is, in fact, the patient's increasingly successful functioning and integration into the natural environment that is the hoped-for, final stage of successful rehabilitation.

The prognosis for an individual's rehabilitation, in terms of both the extent of independent functioning regained and the time required to achieve it, cannot be predicted with precision. Rather, the prognosis for a given medical condition typically is a statistical description of how other patients with similar conditions have fared in the past. Thus, for example, we know that the first three or four months following a stroke (cerebrovascular accident) is the period when the greatest improvement takes place (both spontaneously and in response to treatment) and which usually foreshadows the rate and extent of further recovery. We know that following traumatic head injury, younger patients and probably those with shorter comas at the time of injury tend to do better. We know also, however, that a person who has sustained a head injury may show surprising neurologic and behavioral improvement over a period of many years. Two instances of injury or disease are rarely identical, however, and certainly no two people or their life situations are the same. Thus, the course and duration of rehabilitation differ widely among patients, and prognoses remain frustratingly elusive. Only the general goals of rehabilitation are stable over time and among individuals; namely, the achievement of *optimal* physical, personal, and social functioning.

# 2 Coping with Chronic Disability

Chronic disability refers to a long-term impairment that results from the organic compromise associated with either disease or injury. Disabling chronic illness includes a wide range of conditions, such as cerebrovascular disease (e.g., stroke, arteriosclerosis), neurologic disease (e.g., multiple sclerosis, Parkinson's disease), renal failure, pulmonary disease, arthritis, diabetes, and coronary diseases. Common disabling injuries include spinal-cord compromise, traumatic head injury, damage to sensory apparatus (ear or eye injuries), limb amputations, and burns.

The course of chronic disease or traumatic injury can be viewed in terms of both objective, external events (what can be observed to happen to a person) and the subjective experience of the person involved (how the person perceives, interprets, and responds to the events). Our understanding of the patient's behavior can be facilitated by our learning to recognize the typical characteristics of each of these processes during rehabilitation. This understanding, in turn, should enhance our ability to choose therapeutic strategies appropriate to the patient's psychological and medical condition.

## The Objective Course of Events

There are objective stages in the process of learning to live with a disabling disease of gradual onset; namely, the appearance of symptoms, medical consultation, evaluation and diagnosis, treatment, and rehabilitation. The course of events associated with medical crises, such as an acute disease process or injury, varies somewhat from those associated with diseases of slow onset. In acute cases, the onset of disability is totally unforeseen and has not been foreshadowed by symptoms; thus, medical consultation, evaluation, and diagnosis are initiated abruptly, immediately following the crisis, and are followed by treatment and rehabilitation, as needed.

In *nonprogressive conditions* (those in which organic deficits are not expected to worsen), the patient's functioning is expected to improve from maximal impairment, sometime during acute care, to optimal recovery of functioning. Rehabilitation may continue over an extended period of time, but is expected to produce progressive recovery without the appearance of additional deficits that impede progress or cause regresssion. Consider, for example, the case of a 23-year-old woman who noticed increasingly severe headaches and intermittent weakness in her right arm and leg over a period of several months (appearance of symptoms). She presented her concerns to her family physician and a neurologist (medical consultation). A full physical and neurological examination, blood tests, and CAT scan of her brain were performed, and a left-hemisphere aneurysm was identified (diagnosis). Surgical intervention was recommended and accomplished successfully (treatment). Medical follow up and rehabilitation, primarily to improve strength and coordination of her right side, were initiated (rehabilitation). Nine months following surgery, the woman was back at work half time and managing her household, independently, with minimal residual problems. She continued exercises at home and planned to return to full-time work and resume participation in previously enjoyed sports. Complications from her aneurysm were not expected.

In *progressive conditions* (those in which organic deficits are expected to worsen, as with metastatic cancer, multiple sclerosis, or Huntington's chorea), the course of disability-related events continues beyond initial treatment and rehabilitation. It includes remissions and exacerbations of the disease; further treatment and rehabilitation; and, in terminal conditions, death.

An example here would be a 32-year-old man who was given the diagnosis of a brain tumor in his left frontal lobe (see Chapter 9). He underwent surgery for removal of the tumor, followed by radiation therapy to deter further regrowth (treatment). He tolerated these procedures well and returned to nearly full functioning at home and at work (remission of symptoms). One year later, he noticed the recurrence of severe headaches, the appearance of speech difficulties, and right hemiparesis (relapse). Following medical reevaluation, further radiation and chemotherapy were initated, as were speech, occupational, and physical therapies (treatment and rehabilitation). Personal and family counseling were initiated to help the patient and his family cope with his dreaded deterioration. Following two further remissions and exacerbations of the disease during the next two years, the patient's functioning declined markedly and death became imminent. With medication, the patient was helped to remain reasonably comfortable at home, while both he and his family engaged in religious and psychological counseling in preparation for his death (the terminal stage).

## The Subjective Responses to Illness and Injury

The emotional and cognitive reactions experienced by patients who confront illness or injury are, by their nature, less uniform, clearly observable, and predictable than are the objective events just described. Although certain responses are typical, stages of emotional reaction are not discrete and do not follow a rigid or unidirectional course. A sketch can be given, however, of the psychological processes generally associated with a patient's progression from the onset of symptoms (or injury) to successful adjustment with rehabilitation. This provides a framework for the preliminary assessment of a patient's psychological status.

*Ambivalence.* During the early stages of disease, a person often experiences ambivalence in recognizing the serious nature of symptoms and in seeking medical attention. The person may vacillate between being aware of symptoms and feeling symptom free, between interpreting signs of disease as serious and as relatively benign. The person is likely to alternate between periods of acute sensitivity to symptoms and anxiety regarding their meaning, and periods of inattention to symptoms and denial of their potential ramifications.

Moreover, once symptoms are recognized as serious, the person may vacillate between wanting to seek medical attention as a means of cure, and wanting to avoid medical treatment in order to avoid the confirmation of disease. The patient may wish to avoid having to undergo feared, painful treatment, or having to hear a poor prognosis. At some point, however, the person finally seeks professional consultation due to increasingly severe symptoms, or finds himself under medical care as the result of an acute crisis.

*Shock and Denial.* Following the evaluation and diagnosis of a severe disease or of deficits resulting from injury, a patient frequently experiences feelings of disbelief, emotional numbness, and depersonalization ("I don't feel like this is happening to *me*"). These experiences reflect the patient's psychological defense against accepting information that would be emotionally overwhelming, and thus intellectually and psychologically debilitating, if confronted in its entirety at that time. During this initial period, the person takes in and processes only limited amounts of information, and often has restricted problem-solving abilities. His affect and planning typically are grossly unrealistic in view of likely possibilities.

*Initial Coping.* Following a period of shock and global denial, patients typically begin to cope in a manner consistent with their premorbid behavioral styles, sometimes in exaggerated form. For example, an individual who previously reacted to stress by denying or minimizing its serious and debilitating aspects probably will attempt to deal similarly with disability. Such a person may seek little information about her diagnosis and prognosis, busy herself with other matters, and reveal little emotional response. Similarly, an individual who previously responded to stress by intellectualizing may immerse himself in reading and research about his diagnosis, become an expert on his condition, and deal with the situation primarily on an intellectual, rather than an emotional, level.

*Depression and/or Anxiety.*  When a patient's typical coping strategies are exhausted or inadequate to deal with the prevailing situation, there may be resulting periods of emotional distress, most likely anxiety and/or depression. These reactions reflect appropriate recognition, as opposed to denial, of catastrophic problems. The emotional upheaval can facilitate rehabilitation by stimulating the patient's reevaluation of his circumstances and, as appropriate, by stimulating a change to behavior that meets the demands of the situation.

Behaviors that are secondary to or associated with depression and anxiety, such as dependency, self-centeredness, complaining, and anger, also may appear at this time. Grief reactions, in particular, are an important facet of many patients' depression. During grieving, patients focus on and emotionally acknowledge losses. Examples include loss of a body part, specific abilities, attractiveness, special roles (familial, sexual, vocational), or, at the extreme, the prospect for continued life itself. Often, the patient's mourning of losses allows "disengagement" or the "giving up" of lost assets which, in turn, allows the patient to attend to and develop remaining capabilities.

*Alternating Approach and Avoidance.*  When the patient becomes aware of threatening aspects of chronic disability (poor prognosis, loss of functioning, loss of attractiveness, pain), she may be seen acknowledging and then denying deficits; that is, she may approach and then avoid the issues of disability and the practical steps in rehabilitation. Periods of active problem solving and hopefulness (approach) alternate with periods of withdrawal, depression, and giving up (avoidance). This pattern of behavior can be viewed as adaptive insofar as it allows the patient to confront stressful situations in manageable doses and to retreat when realities become overwhelming. The patient needs to organize her behavior and solve practical problems gradually, rather than to confront too many problems at once and become anxiety ridden and unable to cope.

*Changes in Attitude and Behavior.*  Finally, a patient's adjustment to disability depends on her ability to reevaluate her situation and, as needed, modify behaviors and attitudes that might interfere with optimal independence, achievement, positive self-evaluation, or the expectation of acceptance from others. Some changes in behavior are relatively basic and are even imposed upon a patient as a result of disability; for example, using a wheelchair if legs are dysfunctional. Other behavior changes are more complex and require increasing commitment and compliance from the patients; for example, a diabetic person's following a recommended diet and self-administering insulin, or a facially disfigured patient's participating in community social activities. The more voluntary behaviors often require the patients to risk anxiety and embarrassment in confronting some immediately aversive situations of a social nature. Adaptive changes in these behaviors are critical in the patients' achieving truly successful rehabilitation that includes both optimal functioning and a satisfactory quality of life. For example, most people who are paraplegic learn wheelchair mobility, bowel and bladder care, and information about their sexual functioning. Beyond this, however, are further potential achievements for a paraplegic, such as going out into the community in a wheelchair, attending social functions, trying to meet potential friends and lovers, and being willing to initiate a sexual relationship with someone to whom he is attracted. Changes in the latter behaviors, built upon specific skills learned in therapy, speak to issues of the person's genuine reintegration into "normal" activity; this is the ultimate goal of rehabilitation.

To a great extent, the development of these socially integrative behaviors seems to depend upon the patient's emotional adjustment, attitudes, and values. Moreover, changes in attitudes typically are difficult to establish because they involve reevaluation of deeply ingrained beliefs and values. In rehabilitation, important attitudes often involve feelings and beliefs regarding disabled individuals and the abilities and assets that are essential for life's being worthwhile. Interestingly, attitude changes, in large part, can be approached by (and can be expected to follow) making changes in behavior (or a range of behaviors). In other words, if a person has experiences that are contrary to those his beliefs have led him to expect, he may begin to change his belief or attitude. For example, continuing the case of the paraplegic patient, such a young man may believe himself to be, socially and sexually, an outcast. These strong feelings may begin to change only after he enters several social situations (probably with others' prompting and support), experiences social success, and finds that, indeed, some women are attracted to him. As this man's experiences support ideas opposing previously held beliefs, the strength of those beliefs may diminish and new attitudes may begin to take form.

## Individual Differences

Although the general trends that are seen in most patients provide important guidelines for understanding a particular patient, it is essential to examine each person's unique situation and experience. We must consider, for example, the extent of a person's deficits, the premorbid functions that are disrupted or left intact, the extent of family support, financial resources, and vocational options. We also must consider the patient's premorbid personality and, most importantly, her interpretation of her disability and the meaning she places on lost assets and functioning. Regarding the latter factor, for example, a woman who loses a breast (by mastectomy) may react primarily to any of a number of potential concerns, ranging from bodily mutilation to limitation of physical movement, loss of sexual attractiveness, or feared progression of a life-threatening disease. Thus, it behooves professionals to investigate the private events (thoughts and feelings going on, unobserved, inside the patient's head; see Chapter 3) that influence the person's emotional responses and behavior during rehabilitation. With this information, the most appropriate treatment is likely to be identified.

## Helping the Process of Adjustment

We have described the process of adjustment to disability as one with periods of emotional distress and coping, behavioral disturbance and adaptive change. The extent to which prevailing conditions stimulate and support adjustment determine the course of progress. Favorable conditions are those which assure that the patient's rehabilitative efforts succeed and are rewarded. Chapters 3 and 4 will describe ways in which the patients' interpersonal interactions, private experiences, and the physical environment contribute to such therapeutic conditions.

Of course, a range of factors may result in a patient's *not* progressing toward adjustment and instead showing maladaptive behavior for which special intervention is required. Some of these special, challenging factors will be considered in Part III.

# II

# Understanding Behavior

# 3   Principles of Learning

An important premise of this book is that people teach each other how to behave. It is a common observation that, while we remain basically ourselves, we behave differently according to the responses we receive from others. For example, we may tease a spouse affectionately if he typically responds with a smile and evidence of pleasure, or a quick comeback. On the other hand, a spouse who tends not to see the humor of our remarks, but scowls at or ignores affectionate teasing, discourages that behavior and soon causes the affectionate teasing to stop. We also behave differently according to the situation and to the social expectations which make behavior appropriate or inappropriate in a given setting. At home, we might hug a friend who comes to the door, but if we encounter him on the street or at a business meeting we are more likely to shake hands.

Thus, different environmental conditions prompt certain behaviors, obvious positive responses encourage some of them, and nonrewarding responses discourage others. We can use these facts about behavior to the advantage of our patients and ourselves by planning an environment and social milieu that encourages and rewards the patient's most effective efforts at rehabilitation.

## Behavioral Definitions and Principles

*Reward.*   A reward or a reinforcer is anything that a person finds pleasurable or typically seeks. Of course, the anticipation of getting well is usually the strongest reinforcer for a rehabilitation patient. Unfortunately, for many patients this seems discouragingly far into the future. These patients, therefore, require more immediate reward to encourage them to keep trying, despite the possibly tremendous effort and pain and the dishearteningly small

15

steps of improvement. More immediate rewards can range from a special treat to praise, attention, a bonus weekend pass, freedom to watch TV, or a more active schedule. Charting a patient's progress in therapy and reviewing it with the patient also can provide clear and powerful reinforcement through concrete feedback regarding his improvement and indication of headway toward a goal (see Appendix A). The effectiveness of other reinforcers varies among individuals, according to their tastes and habits. Anything the person typically likes to do with free time can be used as a reinforcer, for example, resting, socializing, or reading. The same goes for anything that the patient is inclined to buy or choose, from a candy bar to new clothing. The attention of others, however, is one of the most powerful reinforcers of behavior, and it is available wherever people are present. This is especially obvious in children, who will repeat with relish any behavior to which adults or peers attend. Among adults, also, the attention associated with praise, a look, a touch, or even a reprimand at times, is reinforcing. This may be especially true for persons experiencing relative isolation and a reduction of typical social activities, as during hospitalization. Additional examples of reward and praise are presented in Appendix B.

*Contingency.* This refers to the conditions of reinforcement, whereby a reinforcer or a reward is given *only* after the person has engaged in a specified behavior (often under specific environmental conditions). For example, the patient may be invited to go to the day room as soon as he has gotten dressed in the morning, or he may be allowed to rest for one or two minutes after walking independently for 20 feet.

*Stimulus Conditions.* Those aspects of the social and physical environment that prevail at a given time are called stimulus conditions. Of course, all behavior occurs under specific conditions, such as in a given room, or with particular people present, or at a particular time of day. These conditions then become associated with, and come to prompt, the behaviors that have been rewarded in their presence. Other stimulus conditions generally prompt the same behaviors to the extent to which they are similar to the original conditions. For example, when a patient develops a range of independent behaviors in the hospital with a particular therapist, he often can perform these behaviors best at the hospital with that one therapist and will do less well with other people in other settings. The greater the extent to which the new situation is like the hospital setting, the better the patient would be expected to function independently in it.

*Effect of Reinforcement.* Behavior that is rewarded (reinforced) is more likely to be repeated in the future, under similar conditions, and behavior that is not rewarded is less likely to recur. For example, if a person is greeted with a smile and praised for promptness when he arrives at therapy on time, but receives no comment when late, he is more likely to arrive promptly. In addition to increasing the likelihood of a behavior's recurrence, reinforcement can serve an informative function; that is, rewards help a person to recognize that the rewarded behavior is considered appropriate (relative to all other behaviors that are left unrewarded) in the given situation.

*Timing of Reinforcement.* Reinforcement is most effective in increasing the likelihood of a behavior's recurrence if it immediately follows the behavior. For example, it is more effective to notice and reward a patient's cooperative behavior as soon as it happens, than it is to wait and praise his generally helpful cooperation at the end of the day.

*Frequency of Reinforcement.* To teach or establish a new behavior, it is important to reinforce the behavior each time it occurs. This is called *continuous reinforcement*. Once the behavior is learned and well established, however, it is most effective to reinforce the performance intermittently, or after several occasions. For example, when a patient shows few spontaneous attempts to speak or act, it is important, at first, to reward every instance of initiation, interest, or spontaneity. Once the patient has established a desirable pattern of activity and interest, he should be praised for perhaps every third or fourth display of initiation, or on a variable schedule. This is called *intermittent reinforcement,* and it tends to produce higher rates of the rewarded behavior and makes the behavior less likely to stop with the cessation of reinforcement. That is to say, if reinforcement is completely eliminated, a behavior that was reinforced intermittently is more likely to continue than one that was reinforced continually.

*Shaping.* This refers to the gradual training of a skill by establishing contingencies of reinforcement for each small step involved in performing the behavior more skillfully. Shaping is particularly useful in rehabilitation because the patient is not capable at first of learning or performing certain skills in their entirety. Performances that used to be routine, easy, and taken for granted may be exceedingly difficult now and require painstaking effort or the endurance of great discomfort. To withhold reinforcement and feedback until the entire skill is perfected would discourage the patient and prevent him from receiving the information he needs in order to master individual steps in the skill. Alternatively, when the patient is taught small steps and is allowed to experience mastery of each as a success in itself, he can learn increasingly complex behaviors at his own pace. He is more likely to be optimistic and motivated to continue working.

When a complex skill is being shaped, it is advisable to teach and reward the patient for accomplishing the final steps in the task, rather than one of the initial or intermediate steps. In this way, the patient experiences the reward of completing the task, as well as receiving any other reinforcement and praise made available for mastering his part. Thus, in the case of a patient who is relearning to dress himself, it may not be possible, at first, for him to put on all of his clothes in a reasonable time; therefore, we could help him to get nearly dressed and require him, as a final step, only to put on his own socks and trousers. We could reinforce him, at first, even if he puts on socks that don't match or doesn't get them on quite straight. Gradually, we would shape complete dressing by requiring him to put on more items, independently, more quickly, or more carefully.

*Nonreinforcement*.   This is the withholding of reinforcement. It may consist of ignoring a behavior or simply not giving the reward that would have followed another, more appropriate, behavior. Ignoring is one of the most effective and easily used methods of nonreinforcement, just as attention, its opposite, is a most effective reinforcer. When a behavior is ignored and not followed by attention (including the attention associated with punishment) or other reinforcement, that behavior tends to drop out of the person's repertoire. The speed and pattern with which the behavior stops depends upon the nature of the reinforcement that initially shaped and then maintained the behavior.

   If we would like to decrease or eliminate a particular behavior, the most certain method is to be sure that the behavior is never reinforced. It is especially important not to give inadvertent reinforcement to the undesirable behavior by occasionally giving in or by giving the attention that is necessarily a part of a reprimand or punishment. Such intermittent reinforcement, in fact, tends to teach the individual to keep on trying until attention, or whatever else he is seeking, is forthcoming. It teaches him not to be discouraged with only occasional reinforcement and is perhaps the most effective way to make certain that the behavior in question is not extinguished for a long, long time. Inappropriate behaviors that are ignored consistently, on the other hand, decrease in frequency and eventually extinguish.

*Punishment*.   This is the infliction of physical or psychological discomfort. Since physical punishment is obviously inappropriate with patients, the most common form of punishment with them is psychological. Psychological punishments may take the form of criticism, a lecture, the threatened loss of something valued, or an expression of personal rejection (a curt response, a sneer).

   Punishment often is effective in temporarily eliminating a particular behavior because a person will stop the behavior in question in order to terminate or avoid punishment. The behavior that was punished, however, typically is only suppressed and is likely to recur, particularly if the patient is not taught other, more acceptable ways to get what he wants. Punishment has additional negative consequences, such as increasing the recipient's anxiety and anger, and thus can hinder the development of a positive relationship between caretaker and patient. Moreover, the patient's negative emotions actually may serve to increase the undesirable behaviors that were punished, if the behaviors themselves were associated with anxiety or hostility (see Chapter 7).

The importance of caretakers' avoiding the use of punishment and the display of negative attitudes cannot be overstated. Although patients are, for the most part, powerless and unable to retaliate in a directly threatening fashion, we cannot expect that they will respond to criticism and negative attitudes in a positive manner or reward the individual who is punishing them. To the contrary, they probably will retaliate by whatever means are at their disposal, even if the retaliation is outside their awareness or unplanned. Moreover, negative behavior or a setback in their improvement may result from the negative emotional consequences (anxiety) associated with punishment or fear of more punishment. The anxiety may contribute to disorganization, poor problem-solving behavior, and either new or more insistent undesirable behavior.

For example, the patient who is scolded for bedwetting may become obsessed with the need to avoid accidents in order to avoid criticism from staff members. As a result, he may request the bedpan with irritating frequency or, due to the agitation associated with the scolding, he in fact may need to urinate more often and may have less bladder control. This may lead to increased bedwetting. In one such case, an elderly, senile man was punished for incontinence. He was left in his wet bed clothing and scolded in an attempt to teach him that he must not have accidents. These negative consequences resulted in increased incontinence as he showed greater evidence of emotional distress. In a different setting, where he received no punitive consequences for soiling, he showed less frequent incontinence, although he was never able to regain complete control of bladder and bowel functions.

*Long and Complex Histories.*   Although the principles of learning are relatively simple, the factors that control learning and performance in the "real world" are quite complex. Over time, many stimulus conditions, reinforcing events, and punishments impinge upon a person and the contingencies that control actions become increasingly complicated and idiosyncratic. Thus, unique histories of reinforcement can be thought of as shaping unique individuals whose behavior can be understood only through knowledge of this history. This information is discovered through reports and close observation over time. Individuals' histories determine what would be reinforcing or punishing to them, and this is something we must know in order to teach new behaviors effectively during rehabilitation. Thus, while behavioral principles hold true for all patients, their effective application depends upon filling in details appropriate to the specific person and situation at hand. Although many specific processes are almost universally valid (for example, that attention, praise, and success are at least somewhat reinforcing), many are not, and individual differences must be respected.

Probably the most variable factors influencing a person's behavior are the private events going on inside the person's head. Assessment of emotional and cognitive factors is particularly crucial to the evaluation of what is influencing a patient's behavior. In turn, this knowledge helps us to decide upon the approaches that are most likely to facilitate the person's rehabilitation (see Part III).

Rehabilitation workers with good behavioral skills will not find simple situations or answers, and they certainly will not apply standard and inflexible procedures indiscriminately. A mechanistic view of people and behavior will not help us to use behavioral principles and methodology effectively.

## Thoughts, Feelings, and Self-Control

From our behavioral perspective, thoughts and emotions are recognized as learned behaviors. Although people enter the world with different temperaments and emotional reactivity, the development of specific emotional patterns largely conforms to the principles of learning described earlier in this chapter.

Unlike other behavior, however, feelings and thoughts are not directly observable. Nevertheless, these inner behaviors are particularly significant in shaping peoples' lives and often serve as potent stimuli and reinforcing events that influence behavior. For example, a person's inner feeling of well-being and optimism (perhaps as a result of a productive therapy session earlier in the day) may make it more likely that he will initiate social activities or follow through with assigned exercises. Moreover, some behaviors, such as doing assigned exercises, may be maintained by a patient's rewarding himself. For example, he might say to himself, "Great; I did exercises that eventually will pay off in progress. I'm really pleased with my perseverance." This is covert self-reward.

Inner contingencies, in fact, are tremendously valuable if they maintain the patient's appropriate therapeutic efforts. Such self-control enables the patient to encourage and reward her own increasingly effective behavior. Because the patient is always available to herself, self-control skills can offer reliable and consistent encouragement (therapeutic contingencies). Therefore, we suggest that rehabilitation workers teach (by modeling, prompting, rewarding, and so on) patients to reward themselves (by praising themselves or by arranging pleasant events to follow good work) and to develop thoughts and expectations that will make their rehabilitative efforts most likely to succeed. We also should help patients to identify negative feelings or self-statements that discourage their efforts, such as a patient saying to herself, "I can't do it." They should learn to avoid negativity that either punishes or fails to reward desirable behavior, such as a patient saying to himself, "Big deal. I took one little step," after learning to take that step over a period of months. Once these countertherapeutic, inner conditions are identified, strategies for their modification can be planned.

Overall, what patients think, feel, and say to themselves cannot be overlooked without great risk to successful rehabilitation. These private events must be analyzed and structured, to the extent possible, to exert a positive influence on the patient's behavior.

## Conscious and Purposeful Behavior

An extensive exploration of consciousness and purpose in human behavior is obviously far astray from the purpose of this book; however, it is important to note that, in our behavioral perspective, we do not consider a person's consciousness or intention to be a necessary part of his learning and performance of a wide variety of behaviors. Of course, we know that people engage in some behaviors specifically for certain rewards, and they can verbalize this pattern (the contingencies) clearly. For example, we may work consciously for pay, respect from others, and satisfaction for a job well done; or we may agree intentionally with a colleague to gain approval, avoid an argument, or speed up a meeting and have it end quickly. We might, however, show all of the same behaviors without being able to say why, and we might even deny motives that appear obvious to others. Thus, contingencies can be operative with or without the person's awareness.

In rehabilitation, too, patients can be more or less aware of what helps them learn, affects their moods, and keeps them behaving in a more or less constructive manner. It is particularly important for health professionals and caretakers to be convinced of this when confronted with patients' inappropriate, annoying, or countertherapeutic behaviors (see Chapters 7 and 8). For example, a patient's excessively demanding behavior may come to be seen as maintained by the attention and social interactions that follow it. The patient, however, cannot necessarily be described as "demanding *in order to* get attention," and should not be accused of such intentions. Similarly, a patient can be observed to cooperate and get along well with therapists who are abundantly praising and enthusiastic, but to perform less well and not as cooperatively with others who are more critical, sometimes sarcastic, and less attentive. Again, it would be unfair to assume that the patient is working in therapy just for praise and attention, or that she knowingly is punishing the more critical therapists by not cooperating and not progressing well in treatment. The patient's behavior certainly conforms to what would be predicted from the prevailing contingencies, but her awareness and control of these behaviors, and perhaps of mediating feelings of pleasure with the supportive therapists and hostility toward the others, cannot be assumed. Moreover, even if the patient is aware of what is going on, this awareness also can be considered a behavior that develops as a result of the reinforcement contingencies.

In general, we emphasize again that a patient's behavior is shaped by contingencies in the environment. Although a patient's conscious motives (those he can verbalize) can, like all behavior, both be shaped by contingencies and function as stimulus and reinforcing conditions that affect other behaviors, they alone do not cause and direct the behavior. Thus, causes of behavior are in the contingencies, while conscious planning and purposefulness may or may not be involved.

## A Behavioral Methodology

The following is the outline of an approach for professional use in teaching and encouraging patients to achieve optimal functioning and adjustment. It should be noted that the application of behavioral principles in rehabilitation populations should not be thought of as doing something *to* the patient, (acting upon the patient as an object). Rather, the ideal way to use behavioral strategies is within a cooperative venture between professional and patient. The application of behavioral principles also should not be used haphazardly. Rather, strategies should be well planned, systematically implemented, and amended to suit changes in the patient's behavior or in the demands of the situation.

*Define the Behavioral Goal.* The overall goal must be set out, as well as the smaller, component skills that must be mastered. First, we must identify precisely what behaviors we hope to teach the patient or which ones we wish to increase in frequency and which we hope to eliminate. We then should analyze the behaviors into small, component steps, ones the patient will be able to learn most readily. For example, if a patient were incontinent, the initial goals would be to increase periods of dryness and decrease episodes of incontinence. The final goal would be of complete dryness and steps toward this goal might consist of the patient's recognizing incontinence as soon as it happens, and calling for assistance; recognizing incontinence when it starts and inhibiting further urination; recognizing the urge to urinate and calling for assistance; and, finally, recognizing the urge and inhibiting urination for increasingly long periods of time until he has access to a bedpan, commode, or toilet.

*Analyze the Controlling Contingencies.*   We must identify the stimulus conditions under which appropriate and inappropriate behaviors occur, as well as the consequences (rewards and punishers) that follow them. This is accomplished primarily by observing behavior and the associated environmental events and by listening to the patient's report of private events. This information allows us to recognize the contingencies that help to control the patient's more and less desirable behaviors. We then can alter contingencies, as necessary, to shape increasingly adaptive behavior.

*Shape the Desired Behavior.*   Using the behaviors identified as steps toward a given goal, we must start shaping behavior at the level where the patient performs successfully. Next, we can begin to reward her for increasingly more skillful performances. In the previous example of helping a patient to achieve continence, rewards would be given for efforts toward, and then mastery of, successive steps on the way to complete dryness. Abundant praise, in addition to the absence of wet bedclothes, should be reinforcing. Charts and graphs could be used to show the patient that she is making progress, and how rapidly. We could chart, for example, the number of times the patient correctly recognized that she needed to use the toilet, or the number of dry hours.

*Use Reinforcement and Nonreinforcement.*   Reward only behaviors to be encouraged, and ignore (do not reinforce) behaviors that are incompatible with the established goal. It is important to (1) observe whether rewarding events inadvertently follow undesirable behaviors and (2) be sure that they follow only behaviors that are to be increased or maintained. Also, we must reward behaviors that are incompatible with behaviors designated for elimination. For example, it is helpful to praise the patient for cooperation when negativism is to be discouraged and to reward quiet speaking if agitated screaming is to be eliminated. In addition to assuring that desirable behaviors are rewarded, we must be careful to ignore consistently, and offer no rewards for, specified, undesirable behaviors that may interfere with the patient's development of appropriate behaviors. Undesirable behaviors would include, for example, petty complaining, temper outbursts, noncooperation, and negativism.

*Maintain a Constructive Attitude.*   Do not punish, criticize, threaten, or behave in a condescending or belittling manner toward the patient. Such aversive conditions rarely help the patient modify undesirable behavior and often contribute to the patient's development of negative feelings about himself and others. This, in turn, can prompt even less adaptive behaviors that are associated with negative feelings.

*Adjust the Plan of Treatment.*   In any learning situation, we must assess
continually the learner's level of performance and readiness to attempt more
advanced (more independent or skillful) performances. Thus, as the patient
achieves one level of skill, conditions and contingencies must be altered to
stimulate and support behavior at the next higher level of difficulty. For
example, when the nonambulatory patient can balance readily with support,
we should begin to reinforce and praise her for attempts to balance and stand
unsupported and should gradually eliminate reinforcement for standing with
supports.

*Teach Self-Help Skills.*   It can be extremely helpful to teach patients directly
how to set appropriate (attainable) goals, identify steps to be mastered toward
more difficult goals, and arrange social and physical conditions to reward their
best efforts and increasingly desirable behaviors. Having the patient encourage, prompt, and praise his own appropriate behavior assures that a salient
part of the person's environment—his own thoughts—will be available consistently to support optimal functioning.

# 4 Making It Possible

## Environments, Aids, and Devices

We have stated in earlier chapters that rehabilitation is a learning process and that the success of learning depends in large part upon (1) the conditions under which the learned behaviors are to be performed and (2) the consequences (reinforcement, punishment) following the learner's more and less appropriate attempts. In the last chapter, we described ways in which social, interpersonal, and private events influence these factors and shape learning. In this chapter, we present ways in which the physical environment can be arranged to facilitate learning and allow optimal independence to individuals who have a range of disabilities.

## Altering the Environment and Using Aids

People all around us arrange their environments to suit their personal characteristics and abilities and to maximize the effectiveness of their efforts. For example, a tall man buys an extra-long bed and a roomy car to avoid feeling cramped; a dieter empties the house of tempting foods to increase the likelihood of eating properly; and a person lives close to work or to a bus line if he has no independent means of transportation. People also use aids and special equipment to ease strenuous work or supplement their abilities. For example, most people who buy heavy cars opt for power steering; a man with poor vision wears glasses; a person uses a shopping list when going to the grocery store to buy more items than he can remember; and a runner with poor foot arches wears orthopedic shoes. During rehabilitation, patients can use the same practical approaches for accomplishing tasks that they otherwise could not do, or for performing jobs with significantly greater ease. Two such approaches are:

1.  To design convenient and therapeutic environments.
2.  To use aids and adaptive equipment.

An important characteristic of adaptive equipment and good (helpful) learning environments is that they are designed to accommodate the patient's current level of ability and therefore allow the person to experience success and to manage as independently as possible. This naturally reinforcing situation encourages the patient's efforts toward independence and increases the likelihood that she will attempt tasks at the next level of difficulty. Success in an increasingly wide range of activities, and especially in those activities nearly always accomplished independently by nondisabled people, contributes tremendously to the patient's emotional satisfaction and feelings of self-esteem.

Either temporarily or permanently, an individual may require special aids or carefully planned physical conditions. For example, a 24-year-old woman with an incomplete spinal-cord lesion from a motor-vehicle accident learned to get around independently in a wheelchair within two months after injury. With time and therapy, however, walking became a reasonable goal, and she later accomplished this. She used and discarded in turn a walker, quad cane, and straight cane. Her ability to manage in decreasingly "special" or restrictive environments (those allowing wheelchair access, or relatively smooth surfaces) paralleled her decreasing need for assistive devices. Thus, when patients' needs change, recommendations regarding equipment and environmental arrangements will require reassessment and revision.

## Therapeutic Strategies

Recommendations for adaptive equipment and environmental modifications will come directly from rehabilitation therapists in their areas of expertise and from reference materials suggested by them, such as *The Source Book for the Disabled*, edited by Glorya Hale (1979), and *Rehabilitation Engineering Sourcebook*, by the Institute for Information Studies (1979). Of course, finding easier ways to do things or inventing tools for convenience presents a challenge to which everyone can respond. Answers are limited only by our own creativity and resourcefulness. The following suggestions, while only brushing the surface of possibilities, provide examples of common strategies for patients with the described deficits.

*Orientation.*  As described later, in Chapter 10, a person who is disoriented may be confused about who he is, where he is, what time it is, or other significant personal data and the meaning of current circumstances. Such an individual's environment should include such orienting materials as a calendar, a clock, and a window (so he can discriminate day, night, and seasons). These objects should be placed strategically to allow easy and repeated reference by the patient. Signs indicating basic personal information (name, age, family members' names) should be in plain view; there should be pictures of friends, family, and perhaps home; and familiar meaningful objects (a blanket, trinkets, a favorite sweater) also should be easily accessible. Familiarity and predictability in the environment, enhanced by regularity and consistency in routines, activities, and caretakers, should aid significantly a disoriented person's functioning.

*Memory*.  A person who has memory problems should not have to depend upon memory alone for tasks that require the recall of information (see Chapters 9, 10, and 11). Instead, memory aids can increase access to needed information, thus decreasing errors and anxiety associated with frequent forgetting. The patient should be encouraged to keep a diary of important daily events, as they occur, and to use reminders and schedules of things to be done. When memory fails, one always can refer to such a lasting record, whether written or taped. Personal records also provide a source of information for caretakers who must check the patient's sometimes unreliable reports. Repetition and consistency in instructions and activities also will facilitate learning and memory.

*Initiation*.  To stimulate action by a person who shows little initiative (see Chapters 5 and 9), activities should be externally structured and routine. Supplies for activities (the newspaper for reading, cards for playing) should be visible, to prompt the person's interest. The rehabilitation environment also should be highly responsive to the person's initiation, in order to shape increasing self-directed activity. Such environments may include a television or radio that "talks" when turned on; a call light or bell that, when pushed or rung, brings a person; instruments that make sounds when played; and, most importantly (as described in Chapter 3), other people who respond enthusiastically to the patient's efforts in conversation and activity.

*Concentration and Attention*.  When a person has difficulty in maintaining concentration, conditions should be arranged to eliminate potential sources of distraction and to focus attention on important aspects of the environment. Surroundings should be designed simply and without clutter. The number of people present (and talking) with the patient should be limited, and he should engage in only one activity at a time; for example, conversation should be discouraged when the patient is doing therapy exercises.

*Mobility*.  A person whose walking is compromised may regain independent mobility with the use of a cane, crutches, braces, a walker, or a wheelchair. Bars along walls and benches in strategic locations (in the bathtub), can offer help and safety to the poorly balanced or weak walker. A leg prosthesis can improve an amputee's ambulation as well as his appearance. "Reachers" help an individual with limited mobility to reach things beyond arm's length. A hand-controlled car makes it possible for someone with lower-extremity deficits to drive and thus to be mobile in the larger community.

If a person uses an aid for mobility, or is somewhat shaky on his feet, environments should be arranged to contain few obstacles and have flat ground surfaces, few inclines or stairs, and ramps where needed. When feasible, it is desirable for patients to live in one-story, compact homes so that desired supplies can be readily accessible. Phone extensions should be available in several locations, and the television should have remote control. When going out, the person in a wheelchair needs to check restaurants, hotels, and recreational areas for wheelchair access and adequate bathroom facilities. If walking long distances is difficult and driving is impossible, the patient should consider living close to stores and a bus route.

Physical and occupational therapists are especially equipped to suggest other ways to maximize the independence of patients with limited mobility.

*Manual Coordination and Strength.* When one or both hands lack normal coordination or strength, a person may benefit from the use of aids in many activities. For example, in dressing, buttons and zippers may be avoided and replaced by Velcro closings or elastic. A closed cup can help the patient avoid spills while eating, and a pivoting spoon can help him get food safely from plate to mouth. Common objects should be checked for their convenience: Is the light switch easy to flip? Is the telephone a push-button rather than a dial type, and has the Trimline model (which needs two hands) been avoided? Are the water faucets and door knobs easy to turn? The list of warnings and "tricks" is endless and probably is known best by occupational therapists.

*Communication.* Of course, the nature of a patient's communication problem (see Chapter 9) determines which aids are appropriate, and it is best to consult a speech pathologist. As an example, however, the person who has severe articulation problems but intact central language skills could benefit from using a nonoral means of communication. The person might use a typewriter, a pad and pencil, or a computerized writing device. The patient with disrupted central language functions, on the other hand, may make her needs known by pointing to pictures on a display board of objects (food) or activities (gardening). A patient with word-finding difficulties may be helped by a list of words, catalogued according to probable word usage (months, occupations, relatives). When reading skill is disrupted, information usually received by reading can be gained auditorily, for example, by audio tapes, radio, film, and television.

*Sensory Deficits.* As is commonly practiced, those with visual or hearing losses can be aided by the use of eyeglasses and hearing aids. In addition, the visually impaired person might enjoy large print or "talking" books as substitutes for regular books, and prefer television or radio news to newspapers and magazines. Messages or mail can be sent on tape rather than by letter. Further, the living environment should not be hazardous; for example, glass doors or unfenced terraces with precipitous drops should be avoided. For a hearing-impaired person, what normally is heard might be transposed, insofar as possible, into visual material; for example, important communications can be written, and news can be read in the printed media. Visual signals also can be arranged to notify the person that a visitor is at the door or that an emergency exists.

Patients with decreased tactile and pain sensation must arrange special environments designed to protect them from possible unnoticed injuries such as burns or cuts. Toward this end, for example, sources of heat should have barriers around them, and sharp or splintering items should be removed from areas of likely contact.

*Sexuality.* As with people who are not disabled, sensuality and sexual expression for disabled individuals are areas reserved for private taste and control. If partners agree on their use, there is a variety of techniques that can increase pleasure and excitement. Many products that are marketed for the general public may suit the particular needs of the disabled. For example, for the patient with mildly impaired sensation, a vibrator may be pleasurable and stimulating. If the patient's motor coordination prevents him from stimulating his partner adequately, a vibrator may be useful again, in this case for the patient's partner. Other aids or procedures may be prescribed by a physician, particularly a urologist, to assist men and women with sexual limitations.

*Recreation.* Physical limitations often interfere significantly with an individual's recreational options. For example, the fisherman and the cardplayer typically depend on two hands and may fear that the loss of one arm's function (following a stroke or amputation) will prohibit either activity. However, fishing gear is available to suit the one-armed fisher, and card shufflers and card stands are designed for the one-armed card player. Special settings, instruction, and competition for disabled athletes also are available. There are, for example, the special olympics for the intellectually limited; basketball and "jogging" competitions for people in wheelchairs; and therapeutic swims organized for those with rheumatoid arthritis.

Occupational and recreational therapists are particularly knowledgeable about equipment, devices, and community opportunities to enhance recreational satisfaction among disabled individuals.

# III

# Special Challenges

Specific Patterns of Behavior

# 5    The Patient Who Is Depressed

Depression is a common psychological problem, one with which nearly all of us have had some experience. Depression is a disturbance of both mood and behavior. Intellectual, emotional, physiological, and motivational factors all play a role.

## Associated Behaviors

In a broad sense, depression may be seen as resulting from a significant decrease in a person's positive experiences (reinforcement). This may include a decrease in activities that are pleasurable and in which the person feels competent, a loss of significant relationships, or failure to meet important personal goals. Other central experiences in depression are a decrease in positive thoughts and feelings about oneself; ruminative negative thoughts; and feelings of sadness, isolation, and helplessness (having no control over one's situation). Feelings of guilt and anger also may be noticed.

A depressed person often shows little variation in facial expression and body movement, frequent crying, loss of appetite, sleep disturbances, decreased sexual interest, and a general decrease and disinterest in activities, particularly those of a social nature. Concentration, memory, and new learning may be impaired; emotions are blunted; and behavior in general tends to be slowed. Some people show increased concern about possible physical ailments and complain of discomfort and pain. Severe depression may lead people to feel like "giving up" and, at the extreme, killing themselves; this may be fantasy alone or the beginning of a plan for action.

A brief description of one patient should illustrate the emotional and behavioral changes that typically accompany depression. The case involved a 32-year-old married woman with two young children. She worked part time as a designer and was the family homemaker. She enjoyed crafts such as macramé and carpentry and spent considerable time socializing with friends. She was seen by friends and family as a cheerful, affectionate, and effective adult. During a routine breast self-examination, she identified a lump and sought medical attention. Within two weeks, the diagnosis of cancer was made and one breast was removed surgically. Although doctors expressed delight in her response to treatment and gave a good prognosis, she showed remarkable personal deterioration during the following several months. As she spoke, her face was quite motionless aside from occasional crying. Her voice was low, with little variation in tone. She avoided eye contact and typically looked at the floor. She reported difficulty with getting up in the morning, disinterest in how she looked, and fatigue throughout the day. She worked on her crafts projects less frequently and rarely saw her friends. Her only ventures out of her house were for grocery shopping and similar necessities. Although she had planned to return to work soon after surgery, she was having second thoughts and procrastinating. She knew she was sad and "not herself," but felt helpless to understand her feelings or change her attitude and behavior. She was particularly distressed by her feelings of isolation from her loving and supportive husband and family. She said she wanted to live and to feel better but that occasionally she saw images of herself driving her car off the road. She felt no control over such suicidal thoughts.

Clearly this woman was depressed. She had experienced profound shock concerning her vulnerability to disease and was confronted with disfigurement from surgery and fears for her future health. Her typically positive self-image of being healthy and attractive had been shattered; she worried that cancer would recur and was overly sensitive to variations in bodily sensations. She felt embarrassed and sexually unattractive with only one breast. She no longer felt productive, and she missed the reinforcement to her self-esteem that had come from seeing her own accomplishments. Because she had withdrawn from friends and family, she was separated from accustomed social support, compliments, and affection from others. Overall, she felt increasingly helpless regarding her health, her future, and her ability to cope.

## Causal Factors

For rehabilitation patients, depression often "makes sense," is a normal reaction to circumstances, and should be expected. The person is no longer acutely ill or struggling to survive and, often for the first time, is faced with physical and/or cognitive deficits and the broader potential ramifications of disability. The person begins to realize that "life will have to be different" than anticipated previously, and there is increasing time and energy to think about dreaded changes. At times, the patient may view herself as "worthless" relative to the person she was before disability, and she may even question the value of continued life.

As may be recalled from discussions in Chapters 2 and 3, many conditions (particularly cognitive factors) that influence an individual patient's moods must be discovered by examination of his unique history, largely through the patient's own report. In addition to unique factors, however, the following characteristics of the rehabilitation setting and process impinge on nearly all patients and can contribute to depression.

*Decreased Participation in Activities and Social Interaction.* By definition, rehabilitation patients are limited in at least some important areas of functioning. For example, certain recreational activities are not possible for a person who is blind, and the logistics of doing relatively simple activities (shopping, going to the park) may be "too much to bother with" for the person in a wheelchair, inasmuch as they require extra time, effort, and equipment. As a result, the person often does less and narrows his range of activity. Such decreased activity typically results in less social contact, lowered levels and diversity of stimulation, and loss of accustomed pleasure associated with accomplishment for tasks completed and done well.

During periods of hospitalization and confinement, reduction in the number and diversity of activities and sources of stimulation are particularly great. Options and choices are severely limited, and the time not occupied often is filled with negative thoughts. Negative ruminations, in turn, lead patients to decline participation in the activities and social interactions that are available. In turn, this behavior exacerbates feelings of isolation and depression.

*Overwhelming Novelty and Change.* Rehabilitation patients experience a great many significant changes, ranging from personal appearance to job potential and ability to care for themselves. During hospitalization, in particular, patients also face an unfamiliar, often sterile environment, a changing staff of strangers, unfamiliar food and routines, and separation from loved ones and from familiar and secure surroundings. The individual's typical manner of coping with stress often is overwhelmed by the number and extent of changes and the new circumstances that require decisions and new responses.

*Loss of Control and Choices.* Particularly during hospitalization, most decisions, from what will be served for dinner to when visitors are allowed or when a doctor will appear, seem (and often are) beyond the patient's control. This persistent lack of control over important or routine events often results in the patient's believing that "nothing I do makes a difference." Such a position of helplessness, in turn, leads to lowered initiative, passivity, and increased apathy.

*Loss of Independence.*   A person who has been disabled often needs to rely on assistance from others in at least some areas of functioning. This loss of personal autonomy, especially to an individual who has valued his freedom and independence greatly and who previously felt uneasy asking for assistance of any kind, frequently results in self-denigration and associated negative cognitions. Often, in the service of avoiding having to seek assistance, a patient will avoid a wide range of activities that would be rewarding and might have led to some improvement in mood.

*Perceived Loss of Identity.*   As described in Chapter 1, each person assumes many roles in life, for example, worker, mate, parent, athlete, or intellectual. With the onset of physical or cognitive deficits, one or several of these roles may be compromised or lost entirely. Thus, the athlete who becomes a paraplegic no longer can jog, ski, or play tennis; and the brain-injured adult no longer may be competent to work competitively. Such losses result in a significant decrease in activities through which the person attained a sense of mastery and accomplishment. This, in turn, significantly alters how the person sees herself as a person, her own worth, and the value of her life.

## Therapeutic Strategies

In rehabilitation, lessening a patient's depression has two major goals: (1) the promotion of physical recovery, which may be hindered by depressive behaviors such as inactivity, lack of initiation, or limited concentration during therapies and (2) the promotion of happiness and life satisfaction, for its own sake. Professionals, family members, and friends all can help the patient manage depression. The following are basic therapeutic approaches.

*Listen to the Patient.*   Attentive listening encourages the patient to speak, get things off his chest, and disclose the private events that affect his moods. The patient's sharing of thoughts and fears that are overwhelming when kept private can lessen feelings of isolation and aloneness. When we listen carefully to a patient, we learn exactly what concerns him, correct any misinformation (or lack of information) that contributes to his distress, and begin to assist him in problem solving.

Patients can be encouraged to talk by means of the helping person's obvious interest, attentive listening, and expressions of empathy and understanding. The listener can show caring by speaking in a warm tone of voice, presenting empathic body language (leaning toward the patient), reflecting (repeating) parts of what the patient says, and giving a smile and touch (if sufficient intimacy has been established). It is important to accept the person's feelings as they are (although you may wish them to be different) and not insist that they conform to your hopes ("You shouldn't feel depressed; put a smile on your face"). Initially, we must let the patient talk about what he wishes and not force discussions that he seems to avoid, even if we believe he would benefit from expressing ideas on a given topic, such as death or sexuality. Such communications of acceptance, combined with the absence of evaluation and criticism, will allow informative and therapeutic relationships to develop.

*Structure the Environment.*   Arrange the environment to be responsive to the person's needs and rewarding for increasingly active, sociable, and positive behavior. Organize activities that are likely to be pleasurable, and gently "impose" them upon the patient until his affect and energy improve sufficiently for him to plan activities on his own. The structuring of activities interrupts, by external means, the vicious cycle of negative ruminations and withdrawal from activity until the naturally occurring rewards in the environment "remotivate" (shape) the patient's independent interest and initiative.

*Encourage Activities That Will Result in Positive Feedback.*   If the patient initiates any activity that is rewarded, the likelihood improves that the person will continue to participate in the activity and perhaps initiate additional ones. Knowing what was pleasurable to the person before he became depressed will help identify what might get the person going (talking, playing cards, being outside, having wine with dinner). When the patient initially takes even small steps toward greater activity, initiative, or variation in affect, it is essential to notice and praise the person's efforts. If possible, arrange circumstances so that the patient experiences success in what she tries; that is, if she goes out to a restaurant, make sure the environment is suited to her special needs, including wheelchair access and appropriate bathroom facilities. As described in Chapter 3, reinforcement of even small positive steps will shape the desired behavior, which in this case is greater initiative, activity, and positive affect.

*Recognize and Call Attention to the Person's Assets and Progress.*   When a person is depressed, he typically focuses on negative thoughts and neglects sometimes obvious (to others) positive aspects of his situation. In this vein, a disabled person might attend to all of his deficits, losses and disadvantages, with no appreciation of his retained assets and strengths. Similarly, the depressed patient may focus on the slowness of recovery and the persistence of some impairments and lose sight of overall progress.

It is important, therefore, to point out those things the patient does well, the personal assets that have remained intact, and the progress shown in rehabilitation. Enumeration of strengths should complement any list of deficits for which treatment is needed. Charting progress (see Appendix A) or keeping a diary of activity also may help to remind the patient of accomplishments that she is apt to overlook.

*Allow As Many Choices As Possible.*   Having to make choices offers the patient opportunities to assert control over the environment and the course of events. This establishes access to preferred rewards (a favored activity, preferred schedule of therapy) and usually stimulates positive feelings of independence and autonomy. Choices can range from those of seeming insignificance to those of great importance; for example from, "Would you like meat or chicken for dinner?" to "When would you like your family to visit?" "When do you think you'll be ready for discharge?" or "What would you like to do during your years of remaining health?"

*Initiate Counseling.*   Counseling by a professional who is trained in, for example, psychology, psychiatry, or social work can help a person identify sources of depression, generate options for dealing with difficult situations, try novel coping behaviors, and discover new ways of adjusting to conditions that will not change. In the context of a nonthreatening, trusting, and confidential relationship, the patient may be able to reveal personal history and current thoughts and feelings that influence behaviors tremendously but are not directly knowable by others. This information, then, enables the professional to advise other caretakers regarding how to help the patient to achieve better emotional adjustment (see Chapter 3).

*Prescribe Medication.*   Antidepressant medication, prescribed by a physician, may be indicated to help a person manage depression. The major benefit of medication, from a behavioral perspective, is that it often relieves symptoms of depression enough to allow the person to get going (participate in activities, sleep better). This increases the likelihood that the person will encounter natural rewards in the environment. Once a few naturally reinforcing behaviors are established, the person is in a better position to change other depressive patterns of behavior without continued medication.

# 6　The Patient Who Is Anxious

Anxiety, like depression, is a condition of disturbed mood and behavior with which all of us have had some experience. For example, many of us have felt anxious before an examination in school, while in the dentist's office, or when preparing for a social occasion with new acquaintances. At times, most of us also have felt a state of restlessness and agitation that did not seem related to a specific situation or concern. Although episodes of anxiety are a normal part of life, they become problematic when they are excessively intense, prolonged, or frequent.

Anxiety is a learned fear response that people experience under conditions that have, in the past, been associated with potential danger or unpleasantness. As discussed in Chapter 3, a person may feel or behave anxiously without experiencing conscious awareness of threat, anticipation of danger, or the presence of specific factors previously associated with threat.

## Associated Behaviors

Anxiety involves feelings of agitation, fear, tension, and restlessness. Accompanying behaviors often are tremulousness, increased muscle tension, sweating (increased skin resistance), and a tendency toward repetitive, often nonpurposeful, behaviors such as the wringing of hands, nail biting, or pacing. Sleeping and eating disturbances, the development of physical problems (headaches, indigestion, skin rashes), and the heightening of pain also may be noted. Anxiety may impair a person's concentration, memory, ability to learn, and flexibility in problem solving, and it may prompt ruminative cognitions of worry and negativity. An anxious person's behavior also may be characterized by a restricted range of activities and considerable avoidance behavior that is designed to minimize confrontation with potentially anxiety producing situations.

During recovery from illness or injury and during rehabilitation, an excessively anxious individual presents particular challenges for health-care personnel. For example, the patient may demand attention and reassurance repeatedly, sometimes directly by expressing fears and requesting company, and sometimes indirectly by calling frequently for assistance or depending on more help than her condition requires (see Chapter 7). He may ask many questions and demand lengthy, repeated explanations concerning his condition and all procedures. He may be afraid of and overly cautious in beginning rehabilitative procedures as soon as they are indicated medically and may resist procedures that he considers dangerously beyond his ability. Further, the anxious patient may be hypochondriacal and imagine fearful developments, for example, that he will rip surgical stitches while doing exercises or fall while learning to walk. He also is likely to interpret momentary sensations as indicative of physical complications such as another heart attack or stroke. Thus, the patient's anxious behavior can frustrate efforts by caretakers to facilitate recovery of optimal independence, and, of course, it produces considerable discomfort for the patient.

The following case of a 55-year-old man who had suffered a mild heart attack while at home alone provides an illustration of debilitating anxiety in a rehabilitation patient. This man had been married for 24 years and lived with his wife and 18-year-old son. He had been a successful, self-employed, real-estate broker for many years, and typically had worked 10 to 14 hours per day, and often six days per week. He also had been committed to keeping physically fit: he went to a gym daily for an hour and a half to work out with weights and play handball, and he jogged three to four miles nightly, after work. His wife described him as fiercely independent, liking to be in control, and exceptionally competent at whatever he did. Following his heart attack, however, he seemed to be an entirely different man. He cried easily, showed trembling of hands and face, had trouble organizing thoughts and following even a simple routine of therapies, and was unable to sleep for more than a few hours during the night. He wanted his family with him continually, and clung to them when they were present. He made multiple demands on his wife at home and on the nurses in the hospital. For example, when alone in his room, he would call for assistance every 5 to 10 minutes, asking for another pillow, a tissue, or a drink of water. He complained of pain, particularly of headaches, and frequently requested medication and medical consultation to see if he was having another heart attack. During therapy, he was hesitant to increase his range and extent of activity and, when encouraged to do so, began sweating, shaking, and yelling that he knew his heart could not tolerate greater exertion. This patient recognized that he was frightened and that his behavior was somewhat irrational and out of control, but he felt unable to cope more effectively. The realization of his not coping adequately, which was so discrepant with his typical style, led to greater anxiety and decompensation (deterioration).

## Causal Factors

It is easy to imagine that a patient might experience periods of anxiety during rehabilitation, just as he might be depressed. In fact, many of the conditions that engender depression for one person may result in anxiety for another. This is true because each individual's temperament and life experiences (history of exposure to and coping with stress) determine his emotional response and behavior under newly stressful conditions, such as hospitalization and chronic disability. For example, a person who always has been high strung (emotionally reactive) and who has had a long history of functioning within narrow, familiar, and nonthreatening conditions is likely to lack the skill and confidence to cope with and master novel and seemingly dangerous situations. The demands of rehabilitation, consequently, might engender significant anxiety.

In addition to unique conditions that may prompt an individual patient's worries, the following aspects of rehabilitation commonly are associated with anxiety related behavior.

*Lack of Understanding Regarding Medical Status.*    Patients typically have little familiarity with medical jargon and the procedures they are advised to undergo. They often have a limited understanding of their medical condition, of their prognosis for recovery, and, at times, for continued life itself. Even when explanations and choices regarding treatment are given, patients typically are unequipped to judge adequately the doctor's advice or to make a truly informed decision. At times, particularly when a patient's experience does not match what he believes doctors have predicted, the patient may doubt that he is being told all the facts. He then may discount all that he has been told and, in turn, find himself even more devoid of a framework from which to understand his situation. In general, when knowledge is sparse, fear, feelings of helplessness, and ruminative thoughts of dreadful possibilities flourish.

*Lack of Predictability.*    During rehabilitation, a great many events are variable and unpredictable, for example, daily schedules, the appearance of a physician, the speed with which caretakers will respond to requests, and the execution of special and frequently painful medical procedures. Of course, the extent of a patient's response to treatment and his recovery of function typically remain the most frustratingly uncertain of all. Such unpredictability means that the patient receives little, if any, warning regarding future events. This results in two conditions that exacerbate anxiety. First, the patient does not have adequate opportunity to prepare for upcoming and often stressful situations, a process that could enhance substantially the patient's coping. Second, without warning for aversive events, the patient may never feel safe from their occurrence or able to rest assured that nothing distressing will happen.

*Novel Roles, Situations, and People.*   From the onset of illness, injury, or disability and throughout rehabilitation, the patient comes in contact with many experts, therapists, and interested others and confronts a wide variety of novel and stressful situations, such as hospitalization, facing old friends who have not yet seen the patient with his impairments, or being at home but able to resume only a few of his previous activities. During hospitalization in particular (as described in Chapter 5), the patient operates in novel environments that lack familiar objects that are personally meaningful and prized, is required to deal with changing staff, and must engage in therapeutic activities that often are not well understood or easy to master. Many patients feel both an acute loss of control over their environment and confusion regarding the behaviors expected of them.

*Social Isolation.*   When ill or disabled, people's social activities typically decrease significantly and change in nature. When hospitalized, this problem is especially great as the patient is unable to continue contacts with friends and family on a "normal" basis. For example, a patient may find herself in a hospital bed alone after 35 years of sharing a bed with her husband; or in a private room with little opportunity to talk with others except during therapies, when asking for something, or when a visitor comes for what may seem like too brief a period of time. Such social isolation results in a lack of the social support and reassurance that could ease her anxiety. Furthermore, when she has limited opportunity to share ideas and worries with others, unrealistic fears may go unchallenged and rigid, unproductive attempts at problem solving may go unaided.

*Anticipation of Pain and Discomfort.*   Rehabilitation procedures can be painful, both physically (stretching tight muscles, exercising despite shortness of breath) and psychologically (fearing failure in therapy, having to acknowledge areas of dysfunction). Thus, repeated experiences of pain and anticipation of future discomfort and disability often contribute to the patient's high state of tension and ruminative worry.

*Fear of the Future.*   Most patients think, at least occasionally, "What if . . . I don't get any better?" or " . . . I can't go back to work?" or " . . . I am no longer sexually attractive or able to be sexually active?" Of course, both the nature of the person's disability and the person's world view determine the specific fears experienced. In any case, as indicated earlier, the greater the extent to which things are unknown (as the future necessarily is), the more room there is for speculation of the most fearful kind.

*Discomfort with Institutions and Figures of Authority.*   Patients have limited power in the treatment setting and tend to see physicians, therapists, and
nurses as powerful authorities who are in control. His "one-down" position, in
the context of the already stressful situation of being ill or disabled, not
uncommonly leads to gross lack of self-assertion. In addition, a negative
history with authority figures such as parents, teachers, or bosses may lead a
patient to feel particularly vulnerable to rejection or abuse by those with
power. Typical reactions are reticence or failure to ask questions, request
help, disagree with suggestions, or seek another opinion for fear of "bother-
ing" the caretaker and risking retaliation or criticism. As a consequence, the
patient may find himself without information, practical assistance, or the
support he needs in order to moderate anxiety and function optimally.

## Therapeutic Strategies

Although, as we have emphasized, feelings of anxiety are normal and to be
expected during illness and rehabilitation, they also demand treatment.
Effective management of anxiety facilitates patients' physical recoveries,
enables them to learn new skills necessary for rehabilitation (which can be
obstructed by behavior associated with anxiety, such as poor concentration
and memory), and promotes general feelings of well-being. In addition to
treatments designed to meet the needs of each individual person, the following strategies should be helpful.

*Listen to the Patient.*   As described in Chapter 5, listening to patients serves
several critical functions. First, it communicates caring and interest by the
caretaker. Second, it allows patients to unburden themselves of worries
which, when spoken aloud, heard, and reevaluated, often are stripped of their
exaggerated and unrealistic threat. Third, by listening to patients, caretakers
begin to learn how each individual patient perceives her situation and attri-
butes personal meaning to her disability and circumstance. We then can
better identify conditions (particularly cognitive factors or generally unobserved conditions, such as family relations) that provoke anxiety and maintain its intensity. For example, we might learn through conversation that a
patient's family has not visited for several days and that she fears their
abandonment; or that a patient on a ward where two patients died recently
may interpret this to mean that she was placed on that unit because she too is a
terminal case. Once these patients' concerns are discovered, appropriate
interventions can be initiated (a call to the patient's family and encouragement
to the patient to ask family members to visit, in the first case, and the
correction of a distorted belief, in the second case).

*Provide Reassurance and Support.*  An anxious patient benefits from repeated reassurance and evidence that medical personnel, family, and friends
are concerned and caring and will not abandon or deceive him. He should be
helped to feel, first, that it is not "weak" for him to cry if he feels upset and,
second, that his fears are "normal." Such support should be expressed both
directly, in a warm and accepting manner, and indirectly, by attention and
responsiveness to the patient's needs. In the latter approach, reassurance and
support can be offered by periodic, although perhaps brief, visits by a staff
member, regardless of whether the patient needs something. As described in
Chapter 5, a warm tone of voice, a smile, a touch, and expressions of obvious
interest and empathy offer great support to patients.

*Offer Information.*  Clear, unhurried explanations of the patient's medical
condition, the rehabilitation program, and upcoming events typically reduce
anxiety. Usually, facts are less frightening than an anxious person's ruminative
fantasies, and preparation, even for relatively unpleasant events (painful
medical tests, a tube feeding), improves the patient's coping. Complicated
information, or that which might be perceived as psychologically threatening,
should not be given just once, but explained on several occasions and perhaps
in several different ways. Patients then should be asked to "replay" what they
have been told and to question anything with which they disagree or of which
they are suspicious. These communications help to assure that patients hear
what is said (and meant) and question areas of continued confusion. This is
particularly important with anxious patients, who may not concentrate, listen,
or recall information adequately and who are likely to distort facts in accord
with their concerns and fears.

 When caretakers share information, they also communicate interest and
respect for the patient. Interest, respect, and candor contribute significantly
to the development of trust and comfort with caretakers.

*Structure a Predictable Environment and Set Clear Expectations.*  Although
patients may continue to have relatively little ability to determine the course
of medical and rehabilitation procedures, they should be informed fully and
able to predict what is coming. A highly structured and routine schedule of
activities; familiar therapists and visitors (and their behaving in a consistent
manner); and warnings, well in advance, of upcoming irregular events (a
doctor's visit, a test, a community outing) can contribute significantly to
greater predictability. Daily schedules should be planned in advance (see
Appendix C). Exercise routines can be nearly ritualized. Demands and expectations held by caretakers (self-medication, completion of independent
exercises) should be stated clearly and perhaps written down. These techniques can provide patients with a sense of security and decrease the anx-

iety that may be associated with "surprises." The patient should have time to prepare for stressful events before their scheduled occurrence and, at other times, be able to relax, knowing that unannounced stressful activities will not take place.

*Plan and Reward Activities Incompatible with Anxiety*.   It is important that the patient be encouraged and rewarded for increasing her tolerance of anxiety producing situations and for engaging in any behaviors that are incompatible with anxiety (describing personal progress, relaxing, socializing). Keeping busy, for example by watching television, visiting with friends and family, engaging in hobbies, or reading, often is helpful as a diversion from agitated worrying. Constructive diversions also are uplifting, in their own right, as a result of the pleasure they engender. Naturally, the more time spent by a person in doing things that are relaxing and pleasurable, the less time she has left for anxiety and worrying. Activities that require the patient's active participation, such as games or social conversation, typically are more therapeutic than are passive activities, such as watching television. This is true because active participation is more likely both to command the person's attention and to allow her to experience success and accomplishment for her efforts.

Patients should be praised and rewarded for confronting novel situations without excessive fear and for showing increasing emotional control and calmness. The patient's behaviors might, in fact, be labeled "calm" or "in control" and "independent" whenever possible ("You really look calm and confident walking today," or "You've been able to concentrate on your book and not become distracted by worries. That's great."). Such praise will not only increase the likelihood of the desirable behavior's recurring, but also will contribute to the patient's positive self-image. Thinking of oneself positively, for example as increasingly relaxed, helps build self-confidence and contributes to further calmness and the reduction in anxiety related behaviors.

*Teach and Encourage Relaxation*.   Time should be set aside for the patient to learn and practice relaxation techniques. Listening to music, visualizing peaceful images, meditating, or relaxing specific muscle groups are common methods for reducing body tension and associated feelings of anxiety. An example of one relaxation procedure is given in Appendix D.

*Initiate Counseling*.   As described in Chapter 5, a counseling relationship can encourage the patient to examine the current situation and to explore personal, social, and environmental factors contributing to distress. With guidance, the patient may be able to confront increasingly threatening or aversive situations while remaining largely anxiety-free. The encouragement, structure, and praise offered by a counselor, along with the natural reinforcement resulting from the patient's success in appropriately graded tasks, facilitate the development of greater confidence and adaptive coping.

*Prescribe Medication.* A physician may prescribe antianxiety drugs when the patient's anxiety seriously interferes with daily functioning and rehabilitation. When anxiety and anxiety related behaviors (sleeplessness and physiological stress) can be moderated by means of medication, it may be hoped that the patient will become better able to develop, at a later time, skills for coping without medication.

# 7    The Patient Who Is
Demanding and Complaining

Of all the behaviors a person can develop when confronting illness or disability, demanding and complaining are among the most likely to alienate others in the environment. They are punishing behaviors. Often these patients seem to become increasingly demanding despite family and staff efforts to be reasonable and helpful. After awhile, family and staff tend to become angry or resentful and may try to change the patient's behavior by scolding or ignoring him.

## Analyzing Behavior

From what we know about human behavior, we can assume that, for some patients, complaining is the most effective way they have found to satisfy needs (gain reinforcement) in the current situation. Some people have a long history of this; others who customarily employ more acceptable methods may have found their skills ineffective in the current situation and thus have fallen back on this relatively unskillful behavior. Similarly, when a person suffers more severe deficits, becomes increasingly distressed emotionally, or is in more physical pain, as occurs during illness and rehabilitation, his behaviors often become increasingly primitive. These primitive behaviors, then, may become the only ones that the patient has immediately available for use.

Although complaining and demanding behaviors often are upsetting to those who work with the patient, it is important to avoid judging or blaming her. We also must maintain a relatively objective viewpoint and analyze the situation by recalling the principles of learning (see Chapter 3). We should remember that personal and environmental conditions are stimulating the patient's complaints or demands and that, if the behaviors persist, they must be bringing some satisfaction or reward (the behavior is being reinforced). To

47

intervene and modify this pattern, we first must identify the needs being expressed and how the patient's human contacts or physical environment may be stimulating or reinforcing complaints. We then can establish alternative contingencies in which the patient's needs will be met while his complaining will go without reinforcement; moreover, reinforcement will follow more appropriate behaviors (those incompatible with complaining). Our goals will be both to decrease the patient's undesirable behaviors and to be certain that her needs are satisfied.

For example, a young man, who was beginning to return to consciousness after severe carbon-monoxide poisoning, began muttering, swearing, and repeatedly shouting demands for water. After two or three drinks, the nursing staff decided he was just being difficult, so they alternately either ignored his cries or expressed irritation by what they perceived to be his continued, unreasonable demands for water. Not wanting to deprive him of water when there was possibly a genuine need, they intermittently gave him water upon his request. Analysis of the situation revealed several factors contributing to the excessive and inappropriately expressed demands. First, the patient's agitation and poor emotional control reflected a pattern of behavior commonly seen during early stages of recovery from neurologic compromise (see Chapter 9). Second, as may be predicted from known principles of learning (see Chapter 3), the nurses' intermittent reinforcement of demands for water intensified the problem behavior by teaching the patient to demand at a high rate until demands were met. Third, the patient's behavior was reinforced both by water (satisfying thirst) and probably by the personal attention and brief social interaction (reducing isolation and anxiety) associated with a nurse's either giving him a drink or scolding him. As the man became increasingly agitated, in part due to the unpredictability with which the staff responded to his requests, attention, social contact, and reassurance became increasingly rewarding. Fourth, the negative and critical attitudes of the staff, which were communicated to the patient, added to his emotional distress; this, in turn, prompted greater demands for attention, support, and reassurance.

Three basic strategies were planned to modify the prevailing negative contingencies. First, caretakers had to remind themselves that the patient's behavior was in part normal for his level of consciousness and that he was not simply being difficult. Rather, his behavior was a predictable result of his mental status and of the environmental contingencies. This helped staff feel less blaming and annoyed with him, which led in turn to their communicating less rejection and criticism to him. Second, staff decided to keep water immediately available and to offer it to him whenever he requested it and occasionally when it was not requested. By this, the patient would learn that staff were concerned about his thirst and that his requests would be attended to on a reliable basis. Third, the nurses planned to visit him intermittently when he was not asking for anything, "just to visit" and to be supportive. In this way, social interaction (reinforcement) no longer would be contingent only upon his demanding behavior. Over several days, the patient showed less agitation and made fewer demands on the nurses who felt less manipulated and annoyed. The growing mutual trust enabled everyone to work together more cooperatively.

A patient's relatively circumscribed focus upon pain as her major complaint is a particularly common and frustrating challenge to health professionals. With these patients, complaints of pain appear excessive in the light of medical findings and persist despite expert medical advice and treatment. The complaints usually are accompanied by such pain-related behaviors as grimacing, moving with distorted posture, taking medications, or refraining from activity. Over the last decade, the behavior of patients with chronic pain has been analyzed in terms of psychological and behavioral processes. Most broadly stated, these pain behaviors are seen to be stimulated and maintained by the patient's interpersonal experiences and the prevailing environmental influences. For example, pain complaints may be associated with stress or depression and may be maintained by the rewards of attention, nurturance, and concern, which are given as a consequence of the pain-related behaviors. Additionally, complaints of pain may be the only excuse that a patient finds acceptable to herself for asking for assistance. They also may provide the only means of avoiding aversive or anxiety producing situations ("I'd love to go, but I just can't with this headache."). The patient typically is unaware of the ways in which these contingencies influence pain. We, too, must be cautious not to oversimplify the probably very complex histories that lead to excess complaints of pain and the associated demanding behaviors. An excellent examination of chronic pain problems can be found in W. F. Fordyce's *Behavioral Methods for Chronic Pain and Illness* (1976). The following discussion, regarding complaining/demanding behavior, also should be applicable for patients whose complaints revolve primarily around pain.

## Causal Factors

In general, we should start with the assumption that *a patient's complaints and demands directly express a genuinely felt need;* that there is some state of deprivation or discomfort that would be eased, or reinforced, by the occurrence of what is requested. We always must listen carefully, evaluate complaints or demands at face value, and check to see if either the source of complaints or the request can be satisfied. Thus, if a patient complains about a too-soft bed, cold meals, or missed therapy appointments, or if she demands medication, a second doctor's opinion, or a beer with dinner, caretakers should consider each complaint/demand as a direct and valid comment on how things could be improved for that particular patient. The request then should be satisfied to the extent possible.

Once staff members have investigated whether the requests defined by the patient have been satisfied or adequately considered, they should contemplate what other indirect messages the patient may be communicating. To understand how complaining and demanding function to serve needs additional to those made explicit by the direct request, it is necessary to examine the conditions under which this behavior appears and the events that reinforce it. The following are several of the most likely conditions under which complaining/demanding behavior follows a hidden agenda.

*Fear and Anxiety.* The patient may be fearful or anxious that something untoward will happen. In this case, complaints and demands reflect anxiety and are rewarded by the reduction of anxiety when another person listens, offers reassurance, and perhaps checks on the patient's specific concern. The patient may be fearful that, without complaining and demanding, no one will recognize her needs as they arise or pay enough attention to prevent fearful things from happening.

For example, polio victims living in iron lungs have been found to be exceedingly anxious and needy of reassurance that staff will notice immediately any malfunction in their machines. A malfunction would leave the patient without breath to shout for help. These patients easily might develop a high rate of demanding, since the demands will be followed (rewarded) by another person's attention and close proximity, which could mean the difference between life and death.

Similarly, a cancer patient who, during the course of multiple hospitalizations, has endured much pain, may become increasingly anxious that she might not receive needed medication in time to avoid great discomfort. Here, fearfulness may lead to increased sensitivity to pain and a decision to start demanding relief as soon as she feels even slight discomfort.

*Need for Contact.* Complaining/demanding may be the patient's best, although least desirable, means of obtaining attention, social interaction, and personal care. The patient may be lonely, isolated in a bedroom, bored, and yearning for stimulation. Often when he is not asking for something, caretakers busy themselves with other tasks and unwittingly neglect him. Inadvertently, caretakers may offer the most attention to the patient when he complains or requests something, while at other times they may leave him largely alone.

For example, night staff in a hospital generally allow patients privacy unless called. The isolated patient, who may be particularly lonely at night, probably would not ring the bell and ask simply for company or a chat. Instead, she might call repeatedly for someone to fluff her pillow, turn her over, get her a drink of water, and so on. In this manner, she gets another person's presence; in fact, when she becomes excessively complaining, she may receive special visits from doctors, psychologists, and nurses. While these professionals try to change the patient's behavior, their presence, attention, and support may serve instead to reinforce continued problem behaviors.

*Emotional Distress.*   Complaints and demands may mask superficially more generalized negative feelings and depression. From this perspective, caretakers should listen carefully in order to recognize expressions of depression and anger regarding current circumstances, illness, disability, and rehabilitation. Picky complaints about the food, temperature, television, and the like often are more easily expressed and more socially acceptable than are disclosures of personal upset, anger at being disabled, or dislike for the hospital staff. Such complaints also may help the person to avoid thinking depressive thoughts and may be reinforced by the escape from more serious worries. Thus, excessive complaining and negativity may be heard when depression is the patient's primary experience.

*Premorbid Behavior Pattern.*   In addition to the immediate function of demands and complaints in the current situation, these behaviors may reflect a basic adjustment pattern that includes poor interpersonal skills, distrust, suspiciousness, and generalized hostility. In other words, demanding/complaining behavior may characterize the person who has a history of reinforcement for maladaptive behaviors. These individuals see the world as unfair and uncaring and believe they have to complain and demand in order to get what is rightfully theirs. Such patients will become particularly distressed and increasingly resentful of an unsympathetic response to their complaints, which, of course, serves to confirm further their negative world view. In such circumstances, complaints temporarily will become louder, angrier, and more insistent.

## Conditions That Aggravate the Problem Behaviors

Regardless of which of the just-discussed conditions are associated with an individual's complaining/demanding behavior, we should examine the conditions contributing to the high rate and/or irritability with which these behaviors are made. First, the patterns (contingencies) of reinforcement should offer considerable information. For example, intermittent reinforcement of demands would shape a high rate of the rewarded behavior and make it resistant to the effect of nonreinforcement (see Chapter 3). In some other situations, perhaps only loud and angry demands, rather than politely stated requests, result in action (reward). In this context it would be true, unfortunately, that "the squeaky wheel gets the grease."

Intellectual deficits also may lead to a high rate of requests, which individually appear valid and socially acceptable, but taken together are impossible to fulfill. The intellectually impaired patient might fail to recall or track his behavior sufficiently to recognize how frequently he is asking for assistance, or even whether his requests have been met already. In addition, lack of self-monitoring, poor social judgment, and decreased emotional control associated with neurologic deficits (see Chapter 9), can result in irritable, rude, or excessively loud and frequent requests.

## Therapeutic Strategies

*Establish Rapport.*   Building caring relationships with patients is one of the best ways to prevent or begin to modify such negative behaviors as complaining. Positive relationships encourage patients to cooperate with and trust caretakers and to express directly, and in an appropriate manner, their needs, wishes, and worries. The support provided by caring relationships also helps to decrease the anxiety that often is associated with demanding and complaining behaviors.

Building rapport, in behavioral terms, means listening carefully and sympathetically, speaking in a friendly tone, noticing and praising a patient's assets and rehabilitation progress, putting aside time to visit, and consistently following through with commitments (keeping appointments promptly).

In response to complaining, caretakers should listen, perhaps reflect the patient's frustration, but be careful not to express excessive empathy or agreeement when this might inadvertently reinforce negative thinking. Instead, we should listen nonjudgmentally, then matter-of-factly describe what can be done to improve conditions and plan to follow through with anything that can be done. After this, we should try to extract from the conversation a more neutral topic (not related to complaints) to pursue and upon which to build the relationship.

*Identify What the Patient Wants.*   Determine what reinforces or satisfies complaints, for patients' complaints and demands express some real need and deserve careful evaluation. If, after directly stated needs (having to urinate, needing medication) seem to have been satisfied, the patient makes continued demands, probably they express a still unsatisfied, underlying, or indirectly communicated request. To identify indirectly expressed needs, examine what the patient obtains most readily by complaining. For example, if complaints are a reliable means of obtaining social support, perhaps the patient is demonstrating a desire for companionship and attention, escape from boredom, or avoidance of depressing thoughts.

In general, ask these questions: What is the patient trying to say? What does she really want or need? Then try to answer the questions by a behavioral analysis; that is, by identifying under what conditions the patient complains or is demanding (before therapy, when no visitors have come, after appointments with the doctor) and what events seem to follow and reward complaining/demanding behavior (attention, reassurance, medication). Also observe whether or not the identified rewards follow the patient's more appropriate, nondemanding behaviors, because the undesirable behavior may be the most effective way she has to gain fulfillment of needs or desires. Talking with the patient, of course, also may reveal private thoughts and perceptions that stimulate demands/complaints.

*Try to Satisfy Patients' Wants Without Reinforcing Complaining.* Patients' requests or complaints initially should be considered reasonable, and caretakers should attempt to respond accordingly. If the caretaker believes the patient's request is inappropriate or already attended to, she should double-check first to be sure and then, as previously stated, carefully observe when the patient complains, what usually is going on at the time, and what seems to satisfy him. Careful observation should give rise to likely hypotheses that can be checked. Staff then can plan how to change patterns of interaction to reinforce the patient's desirable behaviors, eliminate his complaining/demanding behaviors, and still respond to his physical and emotional needs.

When indirectly expressed needs are identified, the caretaker may find it most productive simply to respond to that real need without discussing the identified need with the patient. If the caretaker has close rapport with the patient, however, she might help him to *label* the hidden need and suggest how he might seek what he wants more directly. For example, in the case of the isolated patient who frequently asks for help with seemingly trivial needs, the staff could offer companionship (the suspected real request) by stopping to chat or say hello. This would be done when the patient was not asking for or complaining about anything. Staff members also could tell him that it is appropriate and desirable for him to seek social activity, and they could suggest positive ways that he could do so, such as by calling a friend, eating with others, or asking directly for staff members to visit when they have time. In addition, staff should help to reinforce noncomplaining by encouraging behavior incompatible with complaining. For example, in the absence of complaints, others could remark to the patient that he seems to be feeling better and might like to do some pleasurable activity, or that it's enjoyable working with him, or that his cooperation will ease his rehabilitation. In this way, staff can prevent the patient from "training" them to reinforce undesirable behaviors, and, in turn, they can teach the patient to use more constructive behaviors in order to get what he wants.

*Identify and Treat Emotional Distress.* It is important to recognize when emotional disturbances contribute to patients' relatively insensitive or inappropriate social behavior, such as complaining. Anxiety and depression, in particular, are commonly experienced during illness and disability and often result in patients' needs for reassurance, in their expression of a wide range of egocentric needs and dissatisfactions, and perhaps in their skepticism regarding the likelihood that concerns will gain proper attention. Suggestions for understanding and moderating patients' depression and anxiety are discussed in Chapters 5 and 6, respectively.

Patients' complaining also may be an aggressive and punishing expression of anger and frustration; that is, anger or frustration are the conditions under which the patient complains. If this is so, the patient probably would benefit from identifying sources of distress, expressing these feelings directly, and attempting to solve conflicts. For example, people toward whom the anger is directed, or a counselor, may help the person identify angry thoughts, feelings, and patterns of behavior. When the anger-provoking problems are resolved, behaviors such as complaining, which may be associated with anger, are likely to decrease.

*Respond Nondefensively And Politely.* Responding in anger or ignoring patients' demands without exploring what needs are left unsatisfied probably will not discourage them but, rather, will increase the likelihood of more undesirable behaviors. This will be true particularly if the patients' behaviors are an expression either of anger (which would be exacerbated by perceived hostility from caretakers) or of anxiety (which would be increased by stressful interpersonal contact). Caretakers should attend promptly and pleasantly to patients' demands or complaints, while trying not to give excessive attention or empathy that would serve to reward the negative behaviors. In order to respond appropriately, caretakers must guard against personalizing the patient's irritable style, lack of expressed appreciation, and continued complaints. The development of self-control should help to avoid nonproductive confrontations with the patient and allow staff to gain perspective, analyze the situation objectively, and formulate a strategy for both changing their own nonproductive emotional responses and helping the patient.

# 8 The Patient Who Is "Unmotivated"

When a patient does not follow, or only inconsistently follows, suggestions and regimens prescribed by caretakers, he often is labeled "uncooperative" or "unmotivated." For example, a patient who fails to practice exercises that are recommended by the therapist, or fails to lose weight as advised, may be considered unmotivated to progress. The patient's unmotivated or uncooperative behavior is a serious concern, of course, because he does not do what health experts believe will contribute to an optimal recovery of function.

Unfortunately, when we label a person unmotivated, we make a value judgment, identify the problem as being within the individual, and intimate that she could behave differently if she wanted to. We thus largely ignore interpersonal and environmental factors that have shaped and continue to affect her behavior. From this viewpoint, caretakers are absolved from responsibility for the patient's uncooperative behavior and consequent lack of progress, and she is blamed for behavioral shortcomings. It is usually more accurate, however, and certainly more useful, to examine the patient's behavior within the context of interpersonal and environmental influences, as well as in relation to her unique personal values and motives. These influences will be found to have prompted and reinforced behaviors that may be either more or less productive for the purpose of rehabilitation.

## Causal Factors

*Goal Conflicts.* The goals of the patient may differ from those of caretakers; thus, the caretaker's prescriptions may seem to the patient to be irrelevant or frankly counterproductive. For example, a cancer patient's goal may be to avoid discomfort and to live only as long as he is alert and fully functioning. In such circumstances, the patient might refuse recommended surgery or radiation therapy that he perceives as debilitating. The doctor, however, whose goal may be to extend the patient's life, could view the patient as uncooperative when he refuses treatment. Similarly, a seizure-prone patient might discard medication that he believes to be counteractive to his goal of maintaining mental clarity. The physician, however, whose goal is to control the patient's seizures and who is unaware of her patient's concern, might label the patient's behavior as uncooperative.

*Relationship Between Goals and Prescribed Behaviors.*   The relationship between agreed-upon goals and prescribed behaviors may be unclear; thus the patient may not recognize that the recommended regimens will make possible achievement of those goals. Such a misunderstanding might occur, for example, when it is agreed by all that the patient should learn to walk after a stroke. The patient, however, may fail to recognize that practicing sitting, standing, and balancing, or exercising for general conditioning, are necessary steps in relearning to walk. She therefore may fail to cooperate with prescribed exercises. Similarly, a patient and caretaker might agree that the patient's depression must be moderated. The caretaker consequently may suggest that the patient increase social interactions and other activities but may fail to communicate the connection between this suggestion and feeling better. The patient, therefore, may refuse to initiate or participate in scheduled activities.

*Cognitive and Psychological Limitations.*   In order for a patient to cooperate, certain basic skills must be intact and psychological conditions be met. For example, the patient must be able to understand what is asked of him, remember the directions and associated assignments, and of course have the requisite skills to execute the suggested tasks. To the extent that cognitive deficits and emotional distress interfere with comprehension, memory, and behavioral organization, the patient's resulting behavior can appear to be lacking in motivation or cooperation. Behavioral characteristics such as flattened affect, low level of initiation, and psychomotor slowness, in particular, often are interpreted as evidence of poor motivation, despite their frequently being associated with neurologic deficit (see Chapter 9).

*Practical Obstacles.*   In addition to being able to understand and execute recommended behaviors, patients will need convenient access to requisite environmental resources if we are to increase the likelihood of their compliance with rehabilitation regimens. For example, if a patient is advised to participate in community social activities, transportation and at least some money will be needed. By the same token, if a patient is told to practice relaxation exercises twice a day during working hours, the patient must be able to take the required work breaks.

*Countertherapeutic Reinforcement.* Cooperative behaviors may be punished and uncooperative behaviors rewarded. Cooperation often is taken for granted and hardly commented upon, while noncooperation results in attention and concern from family, therapists, and doctors. Thus, uncooperative behaviors may be maintained by the selective attention they receive, even if the attention is negative and intended to discourage them. In addition, there is a wide range of other interpersonal and environmental conditions that influence a person's behavior; these contingencies are complex and difficult to discern. For example, we might call a patient unmotivated if he consistently visits with others when he should be in physical therapy. We may discover, however, that his nonattendance in therapy is reinforced by avoidance of the physical pain and emotional distress generated for him in therapy. Both the immediate reinforcement of pleasant social interaction and the avoidance of distress and pain keep the patient socializing, rather than going to therapy. This may occur despite the patient's genuine desire for physical improvement, and without his conscious awareness of his avoidance pattern.

*Interpersonal Conflicts.* Interpersonal conflicts that interfere with therapeutic efforts may be specific to the personalities or values of those involved or attributable largely to circumstances such as the relatively powerless position of a patient during treatment. It is important to be sensitive to oppositional or noncooperative behavior that expresses the patient's assertion of power and autonomy. This is particularly likely to happen when a patient fails to recognize therapists' expertise, does not share values or sentiments in common with caretakers, or does not perceive important caretakers as empathic or caring for his needs. Certain patients' social histories may make it especially difficult for them to follow recommendations from particular staff members. For example, men (particularly of older generations) may refuse advice from women therapists, or older patients may become incensed at feeling controlled by much younger people.

## Therapeutic Strategies

When cooperation and motivation are viewed as behaviors that are influenced enormously by external forces (physical and social conditions), caretakers and family members can recognize their ability and responsibility to promote the patient's best efforts in rehabilitation. This entails identifying contingencies that maintain oppositional, rather than cooperative, behavior and then rearranging them to stimulate and reward cooperative behaviors while allowing uncooperative behaviors to go unrewarded (see Chapters 3 and 4). The following approaches are general strategies for maintaining a patient's cooperation and motivation.

*Establish Rapport.* Listen to the patient's concerns, express empathy, and acknowledge the difficulty of his situation. Offer support and praise for therapeutic gains and for all efforts in therapy. In tone, manner, and content, express respect for the person and recognition of his personal history (of health, competence) as well as of his current circumstances. Avoid confrontations and criticism that will lead to animosity and power struggles.

*Agree on Goals and the Ways to Achieve Them.* Caretakers should be candid in describing what they see as the patient's assets and deficits, the goals they consider reasonable for her, and the steps they suggest for approaching specific goals. The formulation of a treatment plan, however, should incorporate the patient's desires, needs, and proposals. When a patient fully understands the steps in a rehabilitation program (and their rationale), she is more likely to follow prescriptions. Moreover, when she perceives that she has had input into determining the nature of her rehabilitation program, she is even more likely to cooperate.

*Make Cooperation Easy.* Making it most likely that the patient will cooperate involves setting clear expectations for the patient, giving instructions (with modeling and feedback as needed) that are easy to understand, and giving assignments that are appropriate to the patient's level of functioning. Practical obstacles (limited finances, the lack of transportation) should be anticipated when recommendations are made, and they should be resolved in advance.

*Arrange Routines and Habits for Therapies, Medications, and Other Therapeutic Activities.* Activities that are scheduled in advance and made routine are more likely to be accomplished than those that are renegotiated frequently. Schedules avoid the necessity for repeated bargaining and decision making where the patient may choose to agree or disagree with the proposed program. Routines build habits that are resistant to the influence of changing moods.

*Reinforce Cooperation.* This may be done by praising cooperation directly or by arranging rewarding events to follow cooperative behavior. For example, if despite agreed-upon goals and adequate explanations a patient frequently refuses medication, it may be wise to offer medication before a meal or prior to a family visit (*if* eating and seeing family are reinforcing events). We can say something like, "I've got your pills here. As soon as you take these, I'll have your dinner brought in," or " . . . tell your family you're ready to see them." The contingency is clear and stated in a positive rather than in a punitive or challenging manner. Of course, we must avoid the more negative and threatening position of, "If you don't take these pills, you won't have dinner," or " . . . won't see your visitors." In addition to reinforcing cooperative behaviors, it is important to see that less desirable (uncooperative) behaviors go unrewarded as much as possible.

When progress is slow or treatment regimens painful and psychologically stressful, it is particularly important to arrange external rewards for compliance and cooperation. If and when progress becomes more apparent and treatment less aversive, the natural and intrinsic rewards of getting better will contribute greatly to increased cooperation.

*Treat Emotional Distress.*   Depression often results in lowered levels of activity and initiation, blunted emotions, and failure to follow through with intentions. The moderation of depression (see Chapter 5) should improve the patient's affect, initiation, and ability to accomplish suggested activities.

Similarly, anxiety results in symptoms that can be interpreted as reflecting a lack of motivation. For example, anxiety often results in behavioral disorganization and avoidance of situations perceived as threatening. Lessening anxiety (see Chapter 6) should decrease such avoidance behavior and promote more active participation in treatment.

# 9  The Patient Who Is Brain-Injured

In order to work most therapeutically with brain-injured patients, health professionals must be aware of the kinds of behavior that these patients usually exhibit and we must be able to discriminate them from similar behaviors of a functional (psychological) etiology. As we recognize that certain behaviors are associated with neurological damage, we feel less bewildered, avoid making misleading personality attributions (and associated moral judgments), and can choose appropriate treatment strategies more expeditiously. For example, when a patient's flat emotional expression, low initiation, and general cognitive slowing are diagnosed as secondary to neurological damage, rather than to depression, further medical evaluation and treatment is indicated, not psychotherapy. Similarly, if a patient's social insensitivity is recognized to be associated with brain injury, rather than as willful crudeness, caretakers will be less likely to take offense and respond to the patient angrily, and more likely to respond in a consistently therapeutic manner.

The goals of this chapter are to introduce the reader to the complex interaction of neuropsychological processes and to describe behavioral approaches for dealing with disturbances in functioning. Consistent with this book's emphasis, we focus on the patient's emotional and characterological changes, which must be managed if we are to facilitate the patient's rehabilitation and adjustment. We also pay special attention to cognitive disturbances that, although not of a specifically emotional nature, can disrupt behavioral adjustment and may be misinterpreted, at times, as psychological pathology.

First, we present an admittedly simplified overview of neuropsychological functioning in the normal brain. We offer this overview as a basis from which to understand abnormal functioning and its associated manifestations, which are described in subsequent sections of this chapter. As we identify impairments, we describe treatment approaches that are consistent with the behavior principles referred to throughout this book.

We emphasize that the therapeutic strategies can improve skills only within the limits imposed by the patient's neurological status. Behavioral programs, when executed in a systematic fashion over time, while not offering magic, can facilitate learning and performance within the range of the patient's ability.

## Basic Neurological Functioning

For our purposes, *neuropsychological functions* will include processes and behaviors associated with cognitive, affective, and characterological responses. *Cognitive ability*, or intelligence, refers to all skills associated with perception, understanding and organization of sensory information, reasoning, learning, memory, and the effective expression or execution of behavior. *Affective functions* involve the person's recognition of her own and others' emotional states, emotional expression, and emotional reactivity and responsiveness. *Characterological functions* involve a variety of responses related to "style," or how the person does what she does. This includes self-regulatory behaviors such as inhibition (versus disinhibition), impulsivity (versus reflectiveness), self-monitoring, self-consciousness, and initiation.

Despite areas of known specialization, the normal brain functions as a complex, interdependent, and integrated unit. As introduced by the Russian neurologist, A. R. Luria, and described in *The Working Brain* (1973), the brain can be thought to operate in increasingly complex levels of functioning. These levels are (1) the reception of sensory data from individual sense modalities (visual, tactile, auditory), (2) interpretation of sensory information (making sense of words or recognizing a particular object), (3) organization and integration of information across sensory modalities, (4) formulation and planning of appropriate responses, and (5) the execution and evaluation of performances. The processes become increasingly complex; as they do, they depend more and more upon a fully functional brain. Clearly, dysfunction in the simplest skill (for example, a sensory function such as seeing) prohibits the occurrence of more complex processing dependent upon that skill (in this case, visual recognition of faces, or reading). Conversely, the disruption of a complex process (for example, planning a sequence of movements), disrupts the effective use of simpler, intact skills (in this case, physical strength or the ability to move).

The brain consists of the cerebral cortex, which can be divided into frontal, temporal, parietal, and occipital lobes; the brain stem; cerebellum; and other subcortical areas (Figure 1). The frontal lobes and anterior temporal lobes are in the anterior (front) portion of the brain, while the parietal, posterior temporal, and occipital lobes comprise the posterior (back) region. The anterior/posterior discrimination is useful in that the different regions

Figure 1. The Regions of the Human Brain.

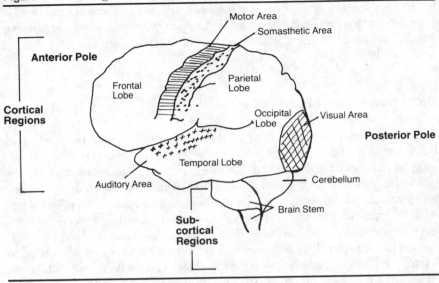

appear to be concerned in several ways with different kinds of functions (or levels of cognitive organization).

The cerebral cortex (and each of the lobes) is divided into two hemispheres, which are interconnected and communicate through the corpus callosum (Figure 2). The right and left hemispheres function in a complex manner involving individual and complementary specialization and coordinated interdependence. For the purposes of this book, we discuss only the broadest and most generally accepted description of lateralized functions, that is, those functions accomplished primarily by one or the other hemisphere.

In nearly everyone, the right side of the brain controls motor functioning and sensation on the left side of the body, and the left side of the brain controls motor functioning and sensations on the right side of the body. Most people also show dominance of one cerebral hemisphere, that hemisphere being primarily responsible for language functioning. Right-handed people typically show dominance of the left hemisphere. Although many left-handed people show dominance of the right hemisphere, most show dominance of the left or a pattern of mixed dominance, whereby functions typically associated with dominant and nondominant hemispheres are represented in each half of the brain. Below we describe the major cognitive and affective functions associated with each cerebral hemisphere.

*The Dominant Hemisphere.* This hemisphere, typically the left, is involved primarily with linguistic or, more broadly, symbolic abilities. These abili-

Figure 2. The Two Hemispheres of the Human Brain.

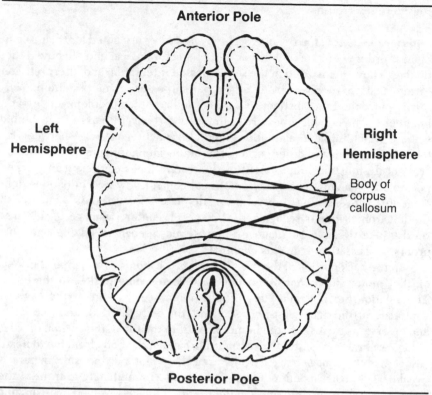

ties include naming objects, formulating thoughts in words, expressing words and organized sentences, recognizing and understanding spoken and written material, and reasoning of any form that requires symbolic (verbal, numerical) processing.

*The Nondominant Hemisphere.* This hemisphere, typically the right, is involved primarily with nonverbal abilities (although it is recognized to have limited language capabilities). Some nonverbal skills include the recognition of visual-spatial material, and the organization of perceptual gestalts, that is, patterns or the relationship between parts and the whole. Familiar skills that require such abilities are using a map (spatial orientation), getting around a building or the neighborhood (spatial orientation), putting together a model, building equipment, doing a puzzle (organization of part/whole spatial relationships), and making sense of pictorial or social information (which depends upon nonverbal cues and details). The nondominant hemisphere also appears to play a significant role in the recognition and expression of emotions (recognizing sadness in someone's tone of voice, showing excitement) and the maintenance of emotional control (inhibiting immediate and inadequately considered responses).

*Anterior Portions of the Brain.*\*   The *frontal lobes* are noted for their role in highest-order cognitive abilities and in characterological and affective functioning. They are involved in the sophisticated integration and interpretation of information received from other parts (posterior) of the brain, self-regulation, initiation, abstract reasoning, and complex problem solving and judgment. The frontal lobes are connected directly to parts of the limbic system, which influences emotions, and also function as the go-between for the limbic system and other parts of the brain. Depending upon the specific areas of dysfunction, impairment of the frontal lobes can result in marked personality changes, decreased emotional control, lowered initiation, deficient abstract reasoning ability, and inadequate self-awareness. One area in the left frontal lobe is recognized as a speech center. Damage to this area results in expressive language problems (see Speech and Language Disorders, discussed later in this chapter).

In the back portion of the frontal lobes is the *motor cortex*. Specific areas on the "motor strip" control movement at corresponding sites in the body. The relationship between sites on the motor cortex and in the body is contralateral (the right hemisphere controls the body's left side and vice versa) and inverse (as the sites in the brain range from the top to the bottom or sides of the cerebral surface, they correspond to sites in the body from toe to head, respectively). Damage to a particular area of the motor strip results in paresis (weakness) in corresponding parts of the body. Immediately in front of the primary motor region is the *prefrontal cortex*, which is involved in organizing and sequencing complex motor behavior.

*Posterior Portions of the Brain.*   Portions of each lobe in the posterior brain function as a "primary projection area" for incoming information, which first travels a variety of pathways through subcortical and cortical regions. Visual stimuli are projected to the occipital lobes, auditory stimuli are projected to the temporal lobes, and somesthetic stimuli (touch, pain, sense of body position) are projected to the parietal lobes. Areas in each lobe interpret their specialized stimuli; however, the areas of nearer proximity to other lobes organize increasingly complex information involving the different sensory modalities. Therefore, the temporo-parieto-occipital region, or "association area," is an area of great complexity and deals with the integration of the more

---

\*Technically, the anterior temporal lobes, along with the frontal lobes, comprise the anterior region of the brain. For the purposes of this book, and to offer a relatively simple and general overview of neurological organization, we describe the temporal lobes without distinguishing the anterior from the posterior portions, and we refer to the entire temporal area as being in the posterior cerebral region.

specialized functions from each of the three lobes. With this in mind, it still can be useful to identify functions broadly associated with individual lobes.

The *temporal lobes* are noted for their role in auditory perception, complex perceptual organization (sequencing information), and memory. The dominant hemisphere's temporal lobe is essential in discriminating speech sounds, comprehending and organizing meaningful verbal material, and learning new or recalling old verbal information (conversation, word lists, stories). Damage to the dominant temporal lobe may result in impairment in any of these skills, resulting in, for example, word-finding difficulty (dysnomia), verbal comprehension problems, or verbal memory deficits.

The nondominant hemisphere's temporal lobe is involved with the discrimination, organization, and memory for visual-spatial relationships and for nonverbal material. Damage to this area results in deterioration of such skills as the ability to sequence pictures that tell a story or to learn and recall sounds, rhythm, or pictures.

The *parietal lobes* are involved primarily in the recognition and organization of somesthetic (sensory) and spatial relations. Behind the frontal lobes, on the anterior portion of the parietal lobe, is the primary somesthetic area, which receives and interprets bodily sensations such as touch and pressure. As with motor control, specific sites in the sensory cortex correspond to specific sites in the body, and damage to a particular area results in impaired sensation in that corresponding part. Sensory representation in the brain also relates to the body primarily in a contralateral and inverse fashion. The large portion of the parietal lobes behind the primary sensory region is an association region and is involved in judgment of tactile stimulation and integrative functions across sensory modalities (touch, hearing, sight).

The dominant hemisphere's parietal lobe plays a major role in arithmetic skill, reading and writing skill, and the comprehension and repetition of speech. Impairment may result in difficulty with arithmetic calculation (dyscalculia), writing difficulty (dysgraphia), reading difficulty (dyslexia), and/or difficulty in expression and comprehension of language.

The nondominant hemisphere's parietal lobe is involved with spatial orientation and relationships among tactile, visual, and auditory stimuli. Impairment may result, for example, in neglect of the opposite side of one's body and lack of awareness of the sensation from that side; difficulty in drawing or constructing two- and three-dimensional designs or objects (constructional dyspraxia); difficulty with dressing, due to poor sequencing of behavior and neglect of half of one's body (dressing apraxia); and difficulty with arithmetic that involves spatial relationships, such as "carrying" numbers.

The *occipital lobes* are involved primarily with visual perception and interpretation of visual information. The primary visual cortex at the back of the occipital lobes receives visual stimulation and allows us to "see." The left visual cortex controls perception of the right field of vision in each eye. The right visual cortex controls perception of the left field of vision in each eye. Damage to areas in the primary visual cortex results in blindness in corresponding areas of the visual field. Other areas of the occipital lobes recognize, organize, and interpret size, shape, and spatial relations in visual material.

*The Brain Stem, Cerebellum, and Other Subcortical Structures.* The *brain stem* is at the base of the brain and connects the spinal cord with the higher cortical areas. It is involved with more primitive and elemental functioning than are the cortical regions of the brain (frontal, temporal, parietal, and occipital lobes). The lowest part of the brain stem regulates autonomic nervous system functioning (functions over which we are presumed to have largely involuntary control), such as breathing and circulation, so dysfunction here threatens survival. The next higher region of the brain stem controls muscle tone and gross, coordinated muscle activity. Dysfunction results in jerky, uncoordinated gait and movement disorders in which the patient has difficulty getting his body to do what is wanted.

A specialized system in the brain stem, the reticular activating system, controls processes associated with wakefulness and alertness, sleepfulness and unconsciousness. Injury to the reticular activating system results in a general disturbance of consciousness, which in turn interferes with all higher psychological functioning.

The *cerebellum* is involved primarily with the regulation and control of muscle tone and coordinated movement. Damage to the cerebellum, therefore, results most noticeably in impairment of coordination, the fine control of movement, and equilibrium.

*Other subcortical areas,* deep within the brain, have critical roles in relaying information among cortical areas and between the cerebrum and other parts of the body (glands, muscles). For example, the thalamus projects sensory input from sense organs to primary projection areas in the brain and has a role in regulating movement (along with other motor centers, such as the cerebellum). The hypothalamus as part of the limbic system is involved in functions related to emotion, sexual arousal, thirst, and hunger. The fornix, malmillary bodies, and hippocampus (along with the temporal lobes) appear critical in memory functions. The basal ganglia, which are nuclear masses at the base of each hemisphere, include regions and pathways for the neurological organization of complex movement, primitive activities such as chewing and swallowing, and some emotional and sensory experiences. Damage to any subcortical area disrupts the particular function of that region, as well as functions of cortical areas that depend, at some point, upon pathways through that region. Neurology or neuropsychology texts can be consulted for more details regarding subcortical areas and their functions.

## Overview of Cerebral Dysfunction

Brain dysfunction (brain damage) may result from a variety of conditions; among them are stroke (cerebrovascular accident), traumatic head injury, anoxia (temporary loss of oxygen to the brain), brain tumor, hydrocephalus (excessive fluid in the brain), neuronal degeneration (atrophy of the brain), edema (swelling of brain tissue), a seizure disorder, neurological diseases (multiple sclerosis, Huntington's disease), or systemic chemical imbalances (electrolyte imbalance).

The kinds of cognitive and behavioral changes resulting from cerebral dysfunction are determined by the interaction of several variables: etiology; site(s) of damage; the diffuse (global, nonlocalized) or focal (localized) nature of deficits; the acuteness of onset; and the patient's age, handedness and cerebral organization, and premorbid intellectual, social, and emotional functioning. Some conditions, such as edema and chemical imbalance, are reversible and, when resolved, can result in the patient's full recovery of brain functioning. Other conditions, such as anoxia and cerebral atrophy, are irreversible and result in at least some permanent deficits. Diffuse damage (or damage to a range of sites) typically results in generalized impairment affecting the most highly developed functions, such as abstract reasoning, cognitive flexibility, new learning, social sensitivity, and appropriate emotional control. On the other hand, certain focal lesions result in more circumscribed deficits, with relatively good maintenance of skills that do not depend upon the specific site of the damage. Detailed examination of the complex factors identified above and, particularly, of relationships between specific deficits and sites of brain lesions is beyond the scope of this book. Such information can be sought from other sources, such as M. D. Lezak's *Neuropsychological Assessment* (1976) and K. W. Walsh's *Neuropsychology: A Clinical Approach* (1978), and from texts on neurology or specific neurological conditions.

The remainder of this chapter offers behavioral descriptions of common neurological deficits (regardless of specific etiology) and, where appropriate, suggests therapeutic strategies. As noted previously, the most extensive examination is given to deficits in affective and characterological behavior. Other cognitive deficits are discussed more briefly.

## Characteristics of Cerebral Dysfunction

Perhaps the most universal characteristic associated with neurological dysfunction is *inconsistency* in abilities and performances. Inconsistency is found in all of the following areas.

1.  Across skills. An individual may retain a superior vocabulary and excellent common-sense reasoning but show significant impairment in visual-motor skills and be totally inept at finding his way around in a new environment. Or a person may lose the ability to read, write, and speak fluently but seems to reason well and function excellently with nonverbal materials. Thus, some abilities are strong and others are weak. No one skill predicts ability in another area of functioning and none reflect overall "intelligence."

2.  Within any one skill area. This means that a person's skill in any one area, such as fund of information or arithmetic, appears "spotty" or shows "holes." Thus, the person shows difficulty with some relatively easy tasks while succeeding at harder ones.

3.  Over time. In this regard, the patient appears unreliable; that is, she performs the same skills well on one occasion and poorly on the next.

These patterns of inconsistency distinguish the neurologically impaired person from the slow or retarded individual whose skills typically are delayed uniformly and are consistent up to a certain level of skill. Similarly, these patterns distinguish the brain-damaged person from the normal adult or child whose skills also usually are developed relatively evenly. The uniqueness of the neurologically impaired individual, compared to the normal child or retarded individual, often is confusing and frustrating for caretakers. It is an essential discrimination, however, for making sense of the patient's behavior and for treating him effectively. Caretakers must avoid treating the patient as if he were a child or a retarded adult. Instead, it is important to attend to the patient's areas of best functioning as well as to his weakest skills: both are informative and neither adequately describes the whole person.

Caretakers also must recognize that the brain-injured individual may not be able to learn via the same methods used with neurologically intact children or adults. For example, a person who has difficulty with dressing associated with parietal-lobe damage will not learn, as a normal child does, by being shown how to dress on a few occasions and then being given repeated practice. The brain-injured person will need far more structure, assistance, and verbal cueing (e.g., "look to both sides of your body") in order to recognize and organize the appropriate sequence of steps. Thus, teaching approaches for a brain-injured person might be designed to capitalize upon the person's best maintained skills (language skills for the patient whose verbal skills are intact but whose visual-spatial skills are impaired), thus helping to provide compensation for impairments.

Moreover, understanding inconsistency is essential for avoiding inaccurate attributions to patients. Sometimes such inaccurate attributions as laziness or poor motivation are made in attempting to account for a patient's performing a given task well on one occasion but not on another or, almost incomprehensibly, failing easy assignments when they have demonstrated mastery of more difficult ones.

In addition to inconsistency, *easy fatigue* and *slowed responsiveness* also are common characteristics of neurological dysfunction. Patients typically need more time to respond appropriately or to solve a particular problem, and their performances tend to deteriorate relatively quickly under conditions of prolonged mental, emotional, or physical exertion.

## Deficits Associated with Affective and Characterological Disruption

The patient with brain dysfunction, like patients with any other problems, may show emotional and behavioral disturbance in reaction to disability and in association with poor premorbid adjustment. However, brain-injured patients also typically show affective and behavioral disturbances as a result of the nature of the injury itself. These disturbances are caused by two, not always distinct, processes. First, some areas of the brain—most notably the limbic system, frontal lobes, and probably the right cerebral hemisphere— have a direct influence on emotional responses. Compromise to these areas often results in affective disturbance. Second, appropriate affective behavior depends upon an accurate perception and understanding of physical, personal, and interpersonal conditions and of behavioral options for responding. Compromise to any area of the brain associated with these cognitive abilities, upon which appropriate behavior depends, can result in significant behavioral disturbance. Disturbances of a primarily affective or characterological nature are discussed in this section, and those secondary to cognitive impairments are discussed in the next section (Cognitive Deficits).

*Emotional Lability*. This refers to frequent and easily triggered mood changes. A person's labile emotional reactions are fleeting, superficial, and appear exaggerated. For example, a previously emotionally controlled man may cry frequently for no apparent reason and become particularly upset at the sight of his wife or the mention of his pet dog. When a person shows lability, however, his emotional expression does not necessarily reflect the true nature or extent of his feelings; thus, the labile person does not always feel sad, or as sad as he looks, when he cries.

It usually is helpful to explain lability to the patient to lessen feelings of being "weak" or a "crybaby." In addition, it is important not to assume that the person is depressed when he cries, and not to delve into and possibly reinforce sad thoughts. Instead, we can redirect his attention to more positive and nonemotional topics and reward his increasing emotional control. Labile patients also report being helped by self-control strategies such as deep breathing or thinking thoughts that arouse anger during times of emotionality. Such tactics seem to interrupt the patient's inappropriate emotional responses by the substitution of different and incompatible responses.

*Impulsivity.*   When a person responds to situations too quickly, with little time to assess her behavior's adequacy or appropriateness, the behavior is considered impulsive. The person "acts without thinking" and does not inhibit responses sufficiently to organize effective behavior. For example, she might begin to answer before hearing a question, or abruptly ask a quite personal question of a relative stranger. She also may speak in a lengthy, poorly organized fashion, talking as ideas cross her mind rather than emphasizing important points and organizing information coherently. Thus, impulsivity may lead to her talking more, behaving at a quicker pace, and showing inadequate social inhibition (by excessive self-disclosure or overly candid comments).

To moderate impulsivity, label the problem for the patient and tell him how others will help him to regain better control. Caretakers should remind the patient to "listen to all I say before answering," and "wait and think before responding." The patient may even be directed to say to himself, aloud, "Wait; think first; respond slowly and carefully." In this way, he may begin to reestablish self-control. Caretakers should praise the patient for going slowly, thinking before responding, and monitoring his own behavior. Be sure to interrupt impulsive responses in a friendly and noncritical manner. For example, in a warm tone of voice a therapist may say, "I'm going to interrupt your quick answers, even though it may annoy you at first. I'll ask you to think first and answer slowly."

*Social Disinhibition.*   Closely related to impulsivity, this results in a person's expressing and displaying responses (to both external and private stimulation) without socially appropriate inhibition and self-editing. The lack of normal inhibitions appears as a disregard for social protocol and lack of social judgment. This may appear, for example, as inappropriate laughter, "foolishness," or such indiscreet sexual behavior as indiscriminate sexual requests or making crude comments.

Despite the neurological basis of the deficit, efforts should be made to shape more appropriate social behavior. We need to identify behaviors for the patient as either appropriate or inappropriate and for either public or private display. Others then should give feedback consistently by praising good social judgment and redirecting undesirable behavior. Fairly continuous supervision for such a patient may be necessary to assure adequate judgment and safety.

*Flattened Affect.*   This refers to a limited range of expressed emotion. For example, the person's face may appear expressionless, his tone of voice sound monotonic, and his body movement fail to reflect stated feelings. To encourage more appropriate expressiveness within the limits of the patient's neurological ability, caretakers can model a wide range of emotional expression and reward all expressiveness shown by the patient (the start of a smile, inflections in voice).

*Decreased Initiative.* This describes a patient's limited spontaneous activity and self-direction. The patient, for example, may sit and do nothing until prompted to action by external forces; or converse little unless asked questions; or, at the extreme, sit in his own urine until directed to go to the bathroom.

External structure and stimulation are important therapeutic approaches for encouraging greater activity when initiative is low. Daily activity schedules should be set in advance (see Appendix C), and recreational materials (books, leatherwork) should be highly visible, to prompt interest. The activities that are prompted at first should be those that will result in rewards for the patient and thus increase the likelihood of her engaging in that activity again, hopefully with greater initiation. Praise the patient's expression of interest and initiation in any conversation or activity, and reward her initiation of appropriate requests by offering what was asked for, if at all possible. These behavioral strategies, along with any neurological improvement that may occur, can improve the patient's rate of initiation, sometimes dramatically.

*Poor Self-Monitoring.* This describes a patient's inadequate self-editing and/or awareness of inadequacies in performance. Such a patient does not monitor and check his own work consistently. The patient may *perseverate* (repeat a behavior, unmonitored, despite changing situational demands) or *confabulate* (include erroneous, made-up material in lieu of appropriate, reality based responses or plausible errors). Inadequate self-regulatory behaviors are particularly troublesome because the patient fails to discriminate good from poor performances and thus does not try, on his own, to improve his behavior or to seek assistance from others.

The most helpful approach with patients who lack a self-critical attitude is to give corrective feedback consistently, to model and then guide the patient's initiation of a routine review of work, to check for errors, and to make corrections as needed. We should reward the patient for spontaneous attempts at self-correction and for saying "I don't know" and seeking help, rather than confabulating. By the same token, a caretaker who knows a patient's reports to be of variable accuracy always should check other sources before acting upon or approving the patient's information. When a patient perseverates, give corrective feedback, praise attempts at self-regulation, and, when needed, interrupt perseverative behavior by distracting or assertively redirecting the patient's attention to a new situation. If the perseverative behavior is motoric (scratching, tapping), it may be necessary to interrupt the movement physically and guide an alternative behavior (put the person's hands on the table).

*Impaired Awareness of Deficits*.    Typically related to poor self-monitoring, this refers to a patient's inadequate insight regarding his deficits. For example, the patient may deny cognitive difficulties, such as a memory problem, even immediately following failures on a simple memory test; or he might show flagrantly inappropriate social behavior and abysmal judgment without awareness that his actions are at all unusual or out of order. This lack of awareness, known as "anosognosia," is different but not easily discriminated from "denial" of a psychological nature.

Although candid feedback and logical discourse rarely will convince the patient, it is important to correct misperceptions gradually, and compassionately offer factual information regarding deficits. We must avoid a condescending, critical tone or persistent explanations aimed at changing the patient's opinion. Rather, we should state briefly the correct information and move on to another topic. Repeated reference to specific deficits, and perhaps writing these down for concrete visual reference, can be helpful. The patient also should be complimented abundantly for all episodes of questioning her abilities, admitting problems, and accepting corrections. Improved awareness, when it does occur, will typically do so in a gradual and inconsistent fashion.

*Concrete Thinking or Loss in Abstract Reasoning*.    This is shown when a person responds to individual experiences rather than integrating many experiences; or when he responds to concrete, superficial (rather than essential) aspects of an experience or thing. For example, in defining "winter," a concrete response could be "cold, snow," and a more abstract response could be "the coldest season of the year, when the sun is at the greatest angle from the earth." The concrete thinker also might have difficulty understanding the symbolic meaning of a saying or metaphor ("a stitch in time saves nine") and might respond only to the literal reference (sewing). Concrete thinking, of course, can interfere with complex problem solving of either a verbal or nonverbal nature, and with the patient's creating a meaningful structure in a minimally defined situation (a philosophical discussion or planning a whole day's activity). Patients who show problems in abstracting often miss the point of conversations, have trouble deriving essential meanings from their experiences, and approach problems in a trial-and-error, rather than in a conceptual, manner. They also may show difficulty changing mental sets; that is, switching their train of thought or flexibly altering their perspective in a given situation.

When talking to a patient who thinks concretely, it is important to avoid abstractions. We should speak in simple sentences, use multiple examples, and not expect the patient to generalize from one situation to another. Open-ended, ambiguous questions (What brought you to the hospital?) should be avoided, and closed-end questions should be asked instead (What medical problem led you to come to the hospital?). Talk about specific events, and provide structure to guide the patient's responses.

*Agitation.* This is a state of behavioral restlessness, great distractibility, and limited concentration and intellectual effectiveness. It is a common sequela of certain brain injuries, such as anoxia and traumatic head injury, and it is typically transitional in nature, as during the period of returning consciousness that follows a coma.

With an agitated patient, the first goal of treatment is to decrease agitated behaviors, such as nonpurposeful, repetitive movements, disorganization, disorientation, and excessive demand for attention. Medication, soothing sensations (touch, music), familiar and consistent surroundings and people, and an opportunity to work off energy by moving about unrestrained (while supervised for safety) often help. Verbal exchanges with the patient should be simple, clear, and highly structured. Treatment should be focused on only one or two behaviors, such as "attending to a listener" and "orienting to surroundings," rather than a range of multidisciplinary goals. Also, learning should be facilitated by the patient's receiving immediate and concrete rewards, such as a touch, a drink, or some valued object, following appropriate responses. Although the use of such rewards sometimes is considered offensive or a form of bribery, it may be the only practical and effective mode of management. Physical and environmental constraints (no access beyond the living area, restraints that keep the person stationary), although distasteful, also may be necessary for the patient's safety. Treatment approaches described in Chapter 6 (on anxiety) and Chapter 10 (on disorientation) will be applicable to the agitated patient.

## Cognitive Deficits

As noted previously, the purpose of this section is to present a general introduction, rather than a detailed or exhaustive examination, of cognitive deficits secondary to brain injury. We will do this by identifying general kinds of deficits (the kinds of functions that are impaired) and those of which we believe it is most useful for health professionals to be aware. We also will point out ways in which cognitive deficits contribute to emotional and behavioral disturbances, and we will recommend treatment strategies.

*Speech and Language Disorders.* Those associated with the disruption of symbolic processing are labeled aphasic disorders and typically are associated with dominant hemisphere impairment. The following are common aphasic problems.

1. *Expressive (motor, or Broca's) aphasia* is a condition in which the patient has difficulty in representing ideas and thoughts in linguistic form. Speech is non-fluent, and word finding and syntax can be quite disturbed. Writing also typically is disrupted because of the central symbolic (rather than the speech or oral) nature of the disorder. Comprehension of language may be mildly impaired but is relatively well maintained compared to the disruption in expressive ability.

2. *Fluent (receptive, sensory, or Wernicke's) aphasia* is a central-language disturbance primarily related to a deficit in language comprehension. This typically impairs the understanding of written as well as spoken language. Expressive abilities also generally are compromised because of the patient's inability to decode language and thus monitor or correct what she, herself, says. The rhythm of speech remains intact but content can be made up of jargon (nonsense) or word substitutions. The patient often is inadequately aware of these speech errors. Some jargon can be understood because stated words often are related to intended words by meaning ("sister" substituted for "mother"), or sound ("snat" substituted for "cat").

3. *Global aphasia* refers to impairment of both expressive and receptive language functions. Deficits usually are quite severe.

4. *Dysnomia and anomia* are respectively, impairment of and loss of the ability to name and find specific words to express a thought. Depending upon the severity of the impairment, a dysnomic person may be grossly unable to communicate thoughts coherently, or may have only occasional trouble finding a particular word. The person's conversational speech may be rambling and circumstantial as she looks for specific words and, in their absence, attempts to explain through the use of other related words and thoughts.

5. *Dyslexia* refers to a deficit in reading and understanding written letters, words, and/or sentences. The patient sees the printed material but cannot translate it into its symbolic meanings.

6. *Dysgraphia* means an impairment in writing. Again, this typically denotes a central-language disturbance and does not result from a circumscribed problem of manual coordination. Inability to write, however, also can be associated with a limb apraxia or a more generalized disturbance in organized motor behavior.

Treatment for language disorders should be coordinated by a speech and language pathologist. The therapist's plan then should be explained to other caretakers and family members, to allow their best communication with the patient and their assistance in facilitating the patient's improvement in language skills.

The speech therapist first identifies the patient's abilities, determining such things as at what level she comprehends spoken and written language (one word? simple sentences? paragraphs?), what method she can use to communicate needs (speaking? pointing? indicating a reliable yes/no to inquiries?), and what her verbal-reasoning and problem-solving ability is. The therapist then tries to teach increasingly more skillful use of language. To ease communication with an aphasic patient, it usually is helpful to speak simply (using sentences of simple grammatical structure), slowly, and with gesturing to complement verbal messages. It is essential to communicate at the patient's current level of ability.

The patient probably will do best in a situation where there are few distractions and only one or two people interacting with him at once. He may need a relatively long time to both understand communications and formulate responses. It is important, therefore, to give him adequate time to respond as best he can and to avoid talking for him prematurely or asking questions without allowing time for a response. Of course, it is not helpful to wait overly long or withhold assistance when appropriate; this simply may make the patient more acutely aware of, and frustrated with, his deficits. As in other areas of rehabilitation, it is helpful to praise the patient's progress and efforts to communicate, whether this involves the use of speech, gesture, or a communication board. Also, encourage the patient to remain calm and avoid too much frustration. This helps decrease the person's anxiety, which could exaggerate communication problems further.

W. McKenzie Buck's book, *Dysphasia: Professional Guidance for the Family and Patient* (1968), is an excellent source for further information on language disorders. Dr. Buck is a speech pathologist who experienced aphasia following a stroke. C. S. Moss' book, *Recovery with Aphasia* (1972), is similarly enlightening. Dr. Moss is a psychologist who also suffered aphasia following a stroke, and his book offers a personal account of his bout with aphasia and rehabilitation.

*Perceptual-Spatial Deficits.* These include a range of disorders in such nonverbal, perceptual skills as visual-motor coordination and the organization of visual, tactile, and spatial relations. These deficits may impair such skills as copying designs, completing models or puzzles, carrying numbers in arithmetic, or recognizing details in pictures or in actual social situations. A specific and related disorder is *inattention and neglect*, which refers to a patient's not attending to one side of her external environment and, often, neglecting one side of her body. For example, a man may forget to shave half of his face or comb half of his hair. Or, when reading, a person may fail to look at words on his neglected side, or at letters on one side of the word; thus, he might read "temporary" when "contemporary" is written. Also, a person might "drift" toward her good side, for example, as in walking toward the right side of a corridor or writing with an increasingly wide left-hand margin. Nonverbal, perceptual-spatial deficits typically are associated with dysfunction of the nondominant (usually right) hemisphere.

Deficits in visual-spatial abilities can be especially insidious because they are not as immediately identifiable as are, for example, language problems. Thus, observers (and often the patient himself) are not struck by the person's limitations and often only feel that something is not quite right. In fact, however, the person's deficits impair his functioning significantly. For example, a patient with left-sided visual inattention is likely to miss visual information that could be critical in understanding a situation. When information is missing, the patient's response may be less than appropriate and, at the extreme, seem frankly bizarre. Another good illustration would be the patient who fails to recognize nonverbal details and social nuances and so has trouble organizing logical sequences of behavior. This individual could have tremendous trouble understanding and making sense of interpersonal behavior and recognizing emotions and communications that are not stated explicitly. Without the aforementioned nonverbal data, this patient, like the one in the first example, is likely to respond in a manner that appears only marginally appropriate or is considered insensitive or confused.

Because language skills typically are intact in people with nondominant hemisphere damage, use of these verbal skills to facilititate impaired nonverbal skills may be extremely helpful. Thus, the patient should have the benefit of verbal cues to guide nonverbal behavior. For example, when a person is dressing himself, the therapist might say, "First put your left arm in the left sleeve, then put your right arm in the right sleeve, then pick the shirt up over your head," and so forth. It is recommended that work and hobbies that involve visual-motor skills beyond the patient's abilities be avoided and that the patient develop substitute interests. For patients with spatial neglect, repeated prompting to "look to the left" and encouragement for the patient to instruct herself to "look to the left" will help. When teaching a task, plan auditory, tactile, and visual stimulation to come from the neglected side, in order to stimulate attention to that side. For reading, draw a red line at the left margin and teach the patient to "keep looking left until you see the red line." During dressing and self-care, use a mirror and prompt the patient to look at her left side and to identify the body parts as her own. She should be praised frequently for correct responses to the therapist's prompts and for independently remembering to attend to her neglected side.

*Agnosias*.  These are disorders in which the patient fails to interpret sensory stimulation correctly despite adequate reception of the basic sensory data (*i.e.*, the deficit is not attributable to primary sensory disturbances). Agnosias vary widely according to the sensory stimuli to be recognized. For example, patients may fail to identify shapes by touch (tactile agnosia) or objects by sight (visual agnosia); they may fail to recognize music or rhythm, or discriminate speech sounds. As mentioned before, anosognosia refers to a patient's lack of awareness of deficits and is particularly obstructive to progress in therapy and adjustment.

*Apraxias*.   These are movement disorders that involve motor planning and the execution of behavior and occur in the absence of primary motor deficits such as weakness, incoordination, and the like. Apraxias disrupt intended and organized movement or sequences of movement. A specific part of the body, such as the mouth or a limb, may be the focus of dysfunction. Ideomotor apraxia interferes with a person's ability to act intentionally in response to a command (his own or another's) or to imitate movements, for example, touching his head, pointing to an object, or sticking out his tongue. Ideational apraxia is the interference with a person's planful organization and execution of a sequence of responses, such as those required for brushing his teeth (picking up the toothbrush, then the toothpaste; opening the toothpaste; putting toothpaste on the brush; closing the toothpaste; brushing teeth).

Apraxias (especially ideomotor and ideational apraxias), if not recognized, can be misinterpreted. For example, when a person does not follow through with an adequate motor performance, she may be seen as not understanding directions for activity, being poorly motivated to do things independently, or being depressed. Such misinterpretations, of course, are most likely to occur when her verbal skills are impaired, and she cannot help to clarify the problem.

*Memory Deficits*.   These can be due to any one or a combination of several dysfunctional memory processes. Problems in remote memory result in the loss of previously learned knowledge, such as one's personal history or material learned in school or on the job. Recent memory deficits refer to problems in recalling ongoing events and learning new material or skills. Deficits in recent memory may result from poor initial attending, poor registration of the material, and/or inadequate retrieval of the information. Material to be recalled may be of a verbal, visual, spatial, or auditory nature.

As can be imagined, a person with significant memory problems can appear (and feel) confused and inappropriate. For example, a person may not act to his advantage because he fails to recall information relevant to decisions. Another person may annoy others with repetitive conversation because she forgets having expressed her ideas previously. Attributions of carelessness or being unmotivated or uncooperative (see Chapter 8) can be particularly problematic and unfair for patients with memory problems. For example, the patient who fails to remember therapy appointments might be considered unmotivated for treatment, or the person who makes consistent errors at work, despite repeated corrections, may be labeled careless, apathetic, or not trying.

If these negative effects of a patient's memory deficits are to be moderated, however, it is necessary that others identify them correctly and help the patient to develop compensatory skills. As described in Chapter 4, written or tape-recorded reminders or a diary should be used to supplement memory and routine, and highly structured activities should be arranged to facilitate learning. Also, verbal memory sometimes can be aided by the patient's using, at the time of learning, visual imagery of the material to be remembered.

If the patient is particularly forgetful, it will not be adequate for caretakers to obtain promises of cooperation, in advance, for a particular happening. Rather, it will be necessary to go through a repeated explanation at the time the event actually occurs. For example, it would be inadequate to explain to the patient that he will have to move to another room the next day because his present room is being repainted. Repeated explanations will be needed, particularly on the day of the event. Similarly, the physical therapist cannot explain once and for all the exercises and procedures to be done. In such a case, the patient may fail to do his exercises between visits due to poor memory rather than lack of motivation. This can happen even though the patient seemed to comprehend fully at the time of initial explanation.

# 10 The Patient Who Is Disoriented or Confused

A person who is labeled *disoriented* is unable to identify his surroundings and his relationship to them. He may not know who he is (name, age, personal history), where he is (the kind of setting he is in, his city, or state), or what time it is (time of day, day of the week, year, or season).

A person who is labeled *confused*, however, shows a more generalized disorientation that disrupts logical thinking and contact with reality. For example, the person may report events that have not occurred, talk of memories as if they were happening currently, or respond to conversation with irrelevant rambling. She may not recognize familiar people and often is not aware of the nature or extent of her deficits. The confused person's internal thoughts and sensations, rather than external (public) realities, assume primary control of her behavior; consequently, her attention and behavior often make little sense to the outside observer.

## Causal Factors

Disorientation and confusion may result from any one or a combination of medical (organic) disorders that affect brain functioning (for discussion of these, see Chapter 9). Functional (psychological or nonorganic) and environmental factors also may lead to or exacerbate a person's confusion. For example, overwhelming anxiety and fear can result in disordered thinking; poorly planned and poorly monitored behavior; lapses in memory; incoherence; and, at the extreme, frankly psychotic behavior involving a break with reality and, often, delusions and hallucinations. Excessive emotional excitement or stimulation also can contribute to confusion for a patient whose neurological functioning or psychological adjustment are marginal. For example, a long visit with many family members, particularly with those who have not been seen for quite a while, may "overload" the patient's limited mental and emotional resources, as may a birthday celebration or a too noisy or visually busy environment. A patient's orientation also can be compromised by such environmental factors as unfamiliar surroundings, unfamiliar people, lack of a routine that differentiates days, little variety of stimulation (as a result of staying in bed or in one room day after day), minimal need for problem solving or critical thinking, and the absence of objects that enhance orientation and awareness of surroundings (clocks, calendars, newspapers).

The environmental and interpersonal events that follow either confused or more lucid behaviors also affect the probability or extent of a patient's confusion. For example, when disoriented behaviors are followed by such rewarding events as increased attention from family or caretakers, a doctor's visit, or perhaps not having to attend a demanding therapy, these behaviors may have a greater probability of recurring. Further, when alert and lucid behaviors are followed by less reinforcement (compared to that following confused behavior), they may have a decreased probability of recurring. Such reinforcement contingencies thus play an important role in shaping the patient's behavior.

Disorientation and confusion can be continuous or transient in nature. When transient, it often is easier to observe what factors tend to precipitate decompensation in a given individual. For example, some patients show increasing confusion, or their only confused episodes, at night. This confusion is likely to be precipitated by isolation and decreased environmental stimulation, both of which typically occur at night. Patients who have variable circulation or oxygenation of blood flow to the brain also are likely to show waxing and waning of orientation. For example, an individual with orthostatic hypotension may show decreased mental acuity as blood pressure drops during periods of sitting or standing but may manifest full alertness and orientation as blood pressure normalizes when lying down. Transient confusion also may occur during hospitalization, as a result of too much change, unfamiliarity, and emotional stress on a marginally functioning person. Typically this confusion clears when the patient returns home to familiar surroundings where stresses are reduced.

## Therapeutic Strategies

The first step in treating the disoriented patient is to identify possible medical causes for the problem by means of physical, laboratory, and neurological assessments. The second step is to identify psychological and environmental factors that contribute to the person's disorientation. Once we know which conditions are associated with disorientation, we can attempt to modify the precipitating (stimulus) conditions, eliminate any reinforcement of disoriented behavior, and plan a structured experience that is most likely to elicit and reinforce more lucid behavior. The following treatment approaches help to arrange such therapeutic experiences and environments.

*Give Orienting Information Frequently.* The person who is uncertain of basic personal data or the nature of her surroundings should be told frequently such things as her name and age, the names of family members, the date, a description of her surroundings, the circumstances leading to her current situation, and names of primary caretakers. Orienting facts such as names, places, and important dates should be posted near her, for repeated reference, as well as in a notebook the patient can keep with her at all times. Although we occasionally may ask the patient some questions in order to ascertain her level of orientation, it usually is better to give this information, because questions may increase the patient's anxiety about her confusion and in turn add to mental disorganization. Giving information, on the other hand, is a nonthreatening way to expose the patient to correct and important facts.

*Provide an Environment that Stimulates Orientation.* The patient's surroundings should be interesting, responsive to his behavior, and a source of orienting information. For example, a reliable clock should be available, and he should have access to a window in order to discriminate day from night. Radio and television news can provide information on current events. A bulletin board of important personal data, pictures and names of family members and friends, and pictures of home or familiar places also can be extremely helpful. The patient could be encouraged to keep familiar objects (a favorite bedspread, a bathrobe, or a long-loved piece of art) nearby, even when hospitalized. Such familiar objects and surroundings often enhance his awareness of personal history and individuality, which tends to increase his sense of security and reduce his anxiety.

*Arrange Highly Structured Predictable Environments.* Consistency and predictability in the environment usually reduce a person's anxiety and help him to learn and remember new skills or information (orienting data, what is expected of him, specific exercises). Daily activities should be planned in advance and made routine; for example, there should be regular times and places for grooming, meals, and therapies. Within a treatment setting, the patient is less liable to be confused if staffing is consistent; at home, also, primary caretakers should be consistent. The patient should be told, in advance, about any special events, examinations, or changes in routine, and these should be explained fully at a level he will understand.

*Talk Simply and Repeat Important Communications.* Sentences should be short and grammatically simple, to facilitate the person's understanding. Conversations should focus on concrete (rather than abstract) and immediately observable events and things. Such approaches help to focus the person's attention, prompt contact with reality, and distract her from internally determined, confused thinking. When instructions are given they should be accompanied by explicit explanation of expectations, modeling (demonstration) when appropriate, guided trials, and corrective feedback. Under these conditions, the person is most likely to understand what she is asked to do and to be able to cooperate.

Since memory is a significant problem for disoriented patients, it is important to plan activities and rehabilitation strategies that do not depend upon the individual's recall. Disoriented people need repeated instructions concerning therapy procedures, even if they have demonstrated understanding of the same procedures on previous occasions. Other supports for impaired memory are consistency in routines, access to written or tape-recorded reminders of what is to be done (taking medication, doing exercises), and limited complexity in task demands (see sections regarding memory in Chapters 4 and 9).

*Do Not Engage in Confused Conversation.*   Although it may be tempting to try to understand a confused person's thinking by asking questions and trying to discern meanings, it is important to avoid discussion (and its social reinforcement) of inaccurate or delusional ideas. Do not attend to confused parts of the conversation, and, if the person can tolerate the feedback, let him know that he is not making sense, or that you think his recall is not entirely accurate, and redirect attention to a concrete and appropriate topic. When a person talks sensibly or gives accurate information, be sure to praise her ("You're really thinking clearly and expressing it well. That's great."). Ignoring confused talk and rewarding sensible talk will help the patient to discriminate between the two, eliminate the former, and increase the latter (see Chapter 3).

*Give Corrective Feedback.*   When the patient offers misinformation, avoid sounding critical or condescending to the patient, but do consistently give corrective feedback. The patient needs to receive accurate information in order to improve orientation and organization of her thoughts. If she insists that her viewpoint is correct, however, do not argue or try to convince her of the facts. Simply state the accurate information and try to direct the conversation to another topic.

*Ease Anxieties.*   When anxiety is one of the conditions associated with diminished lucidity, we must attempt to lower it. By observation and by report from the patient, we should attempt to identify and then alter, if possible, anxiety provoking environmental and interpersonal conditions (see Chapter 6). Familiarity and predictability in the environment, supportive social contacts, relaxation procedures (see Appendix D), and, at times, tranquilizing medication may be helpful. When anxiety abates and the person displays more lucid behavior, caretakers have an excellent opportunity to reinforce the positive changes. Such reinforcement, and the person's own recognition of improved mental status, are likely to reduce anxiety further and to stimulate still greater cognitive organization.

*Treat the Patient Respectfully.* Despite disorientation and confusion, the impaired patient remains a feeling and, at whatever level, thinking person. Caretakers, therefore, should maintain social niceties, to the degree possible, and respect for privacy, independence, and control. Staff members should avoid talking about the patient in his presence, as if he were absent or totally incompetent. Efforts to explain situations, give choices, and engage in meaningful interaction should be continued, despite often minimal responsiveness by the patient. Such respectful treatment is essential for humanistic reasons and because we often truly do not know how much the person is perceiving. An individual who understands only fragments of what is going on may recognize through continued communications that others see him as a person, someone with mental sensibility. This, in turn, can moderate some of his anxiety and can support his best efforts to organize his behavior.

# 11    The Patient Who Is Aged

The elderly patient is an individual who, like anyone else, has a unique history and has learned to value specific ideas, things, and experiences that the caring person must take time to discover. Too often, older people are stripped of personality, sexuality, and style and are lumped together without recognition of vast differences.

Despite their individuality, however, older persons, as a group, tend to show a high incidence of particular characteristics. Recognizing these patterns of behavior, in addition to the individual characteristics of particular patients, enhances the caretaker's understanding of aged patients and facilitates the development of effective treatment plans.

## Degenerative Changes Associated with Normal Aging

*Slowed Reaction Time.*   With aging, people show a slowing of their responsiveness, particularly in motor activity and also in thought. Older individuals take longer to switch to a new train of thought, to orient to new situations, and to organize behavior according to instructions or intention. Movement is slower and reactions to stimulation delayed. Rapid-fire questions, fast-moving and hard-to-follow (group) conversations, or speed-related demands are likely to upset the older person who does not have adequate time to think and respond as she wishes. Under such circumstances, elderly patients sometimes show frustration, emotionality (anger, tearfulness), or confusion. If pressed to respond without adequate time to size up the situation, the patient's behavior may appear inappropriate or, at the extreme, irrational.

*Loss of Sensory Acuity.*   It is recognized commonly that hearing and visual acuity decline with age. Similarly, some loss of sensitivity to taste and smell frequently are reported. A decrease in sensory acuity often results in the individual's loss of stimulation and access to pleasures. For example, failing eyesight may dull the beauty of flowers and make reading favorite literature an onerous task. Similarly, hearing difficulties may exclude the individual from active participation in conversation and may lead to misinterpretation of communication. At the extreme, such misunderstanding may lead to the person's mistrusting others and feeling isolated, rejected, and hypersensitive.

*Decline in Memory.* Forgetfulness and delayed recall are almost universal problems among the elderly. While well-learned skills, information, and personal history usually are not impaired, memory for new information and the ability to learn new skills typically decline. For example, an older individual might remember fewer items of a list or details in a story than would have been recalled in younger years, and he may need more trials to learn and retain instructions for exercises or activities. As is true for anyone, the elderly person's memory may be further impaired by emotional distress associated with circumstances such as illness, hospitalization, or the necessity of taking part in a rehabilitation program. Stress-related interference with memory is particularly noticeable among aged people who already show memory deficits.

*Lowered Endurance and Energy.* Decreased stamina and strength and greater need for pacing activity are changes that almost universally are associated with aging. Unfortunately, it often is difficult to discriminate a normal slowing from the decreased stamina that is due either to relative inactivity and deconditioning or depression, both of which are frequent concomitants of illness, disability, or the narrowing range of activity typically found in older populations.

*Altered Sexual Functioning.* Although the capability for erection, ejaculation, and orgasm often declines in advanced years, the extent of change and the age of onset vary greatly among individuals. One significant determinant of these changes is the individual's history of sexual activity throughout life. For example, a person who has been quite active sexually, over many years, is more likely to maintain sexual functioning during later years.

The amount of actual sexual activity, independent of capacity, also varies greatly among older people. This seems attributable less to physiological changes than to varying opportunity. In later stages of life, the frequency of sexual activity has been found to depend largely upon whether the individual has a steady partner.

Too often, decline in an older person's sexual activity or interest is inappropriately attributed to old age, or is seen as "proper" and in fact is

greeted with relief. A decline in sexual functioning, however, may be symp-
tomatic of depression or a pathological medical condition, either of which
should be treated.

*Increased Risk of Functional Decompensation.* During the later years of
life, neurological functioning changes. Although most skills are relatively well
maintained (except as just discussed) or compensated for, neurological degeneration results in a greater likelihood of decompensation under adverse
environmental, emotional, or physiological conditions. Thus, the elderly
patient is at high risk for deterioration, including cognitive decline, disorientation, and confusion, during periods of change and excessive stress
(illness or hospitalization). Such episodes of confusion can be reversed as
conditions stabilize, or can be the incipient stage of continued deterioration.

An illustration of transient decompensation is provided by an 87-year-old
man who had lived alone successfully prior to entering the hospital for
orthopedic surgery. Although all procedures went well and no metabolic or
cerebral problems were identified, the man showed intermittent confusion
and disorientation for several weeks following surgery. It appeared that
separation from familiar surroundings, routines, and people, plus confrontation with novel information and procedures and his anxiety concerning
surgery and recovery, combined to overwhelm his resources. His condition
improved as anxiety abated and he became familiar with hospital routines and
staff.

Similarly, an 84-year-old woman, who had sustained a relatively minor
stroke, remained confused and disoriented in the hospital and went from
person to person on the ward, asking to be taken home. Against staff advice,
her husband took her home where, within 24 hours, there was noticeable
improvement; within a week her behavior approximated her premorbid level
of functioning. It appeared that returning to her familiar home and routine
and having some responsibility for her own care were significant factors in her
recovery.

## Pathological Conditions

Although the changes just discussed are normally associated with aging,
caretakers must be alert to pathological conditions that also may appear.
When a patient's functional decline is greater than expected, relative to norms
for his age group, it behooves caretakers to identify potential causes so that
appropriate treatment may be planned. For example, when metabolic or
endocrinological dysfunction or hydrocephalus is responsible for cognitive
and behavioral deficits, medical management may resolve the pathology

and, with it, the associated impairments. Old age, alone, is an inadequate explanation for marked deficits and, when used inappropriately, can mask a treatable condition.

*Neurological Dysfunction.* A relatively common neurological pathology associated with aging (besides discrete neurological events such as strokes) is senile dementia or Alzheimer's disease (labeled such particularly when the patient is younger than 65) which results in progressive neurological decline. Common behavioral characteristics are concreteness of thinking; impaired memory, judgment, and reasoning; lowered initiative and planning ability; and weakened emotional control. Several of these early symptoms present a picture similar to what would be seen in a patient with depression. Increasing deterioration, however, which may result in disorientation, confusion, loss of physiological (bladder and bowel) control, and more marked intellectual and behavioral disability, indicate more clearly that a neurological deterioration is occurring. Chapters 9 and 10 contain information about treatment approaches for patients who are neurologically impaired or confused.

*Depression.* This is the most common psychological problem among the elderly. As described in Chapter 5, depression usually is experienced when the number or quality of reinforcing experiences declines significantly below the level to which the individual has been accustomed. For the elderly, reduction in rewarding experiences results from a variety of factors; among them are loss of friends through death or incapacity, separation from familiar environments and family through household moves or confinement (hospitalization), and loss of physical vigor and abilities that previously allowed diverse stimulation. Many aged individuals have narrowed their range of interests as their energy level has decreased, and they have come to place great importance on relatively few sources of enjoyment. For example, it may be especially important to drink a particular brand of tea; to take a bath rather than a shower; or to have a cocktail before dinner, a telephone immediately available to call friends, or a TV set to watch particular shows. Disruption of any of the person's few preferred activities can be a major loss of reinforcement. Awareness of declining abilities, particularly in areas of prior competence, adds to feelings of depression and lowered self-esteem.

Depression is a particularly significant problem for the elderly during periods of illness, disability, and confinement. Threatened or real loss of personal autonomy and dignity is a most frequent source of distress. In the extreme, the older patient who is hospitalized is required to conform to relatively inflexible routines and has to tolerate experiences that violate his values and sensibilities; for example, he may be an alert, up-to-the-minute patient who is placed on a ward with only brain-damaged or senile patients, or he may be grouped with patients who do not share some background experiences, values, or interests.

Too often, elderly patients are spoken to as if they were children (either through tone of voice or through being called by their first name, "honey," or "dear"), lose privacy over their bodies and immediate space (their room), and see decisions being made for them without their consultation. The elderly have been accustomed to making their own decisions independently and to being treated with respect and equality. They have been the caretakers of younger generations and often are unused to being the objects of care and the recipients of orders. Thus, extended time in situations that continually limit choices, and at times are frankly demeaning, threatens the older person's well-established self-perceptions and dignity.

Lack of social contact and support is another prevalent source of depression for elderly persons, particularly those who have lost a spouse, who live alone, who are confined (hospitalized), or who are unable to get around to visit friends. This social isolation results in a lack of incentive to participate in activities and keep intellectually alert, as well as in loss of reinforcement for a wide range of behaviors. For example, without social contacts, reading and staying informed would not be reinforced by active discussion; maintaining an attractive appearance or preparing a healthy and tasty meal would not yield a compliment; and efforts to improve health habits and continue therapeutic regimens would go unnoticed. Overall, without other people, an individual's world becomes frighteningly devoid of stimulation and social reinforcement.

Lack of hope for the future and anticipation of continued incapacity and/or death are, of course, also realistic factors that affect moods among the elderly. Anticipation of prolonged illness, disability, or pain and of isolation in a health-care facility or residence with family (children), where they may feel unwelcome, can result in great anxiety and depression. At the extreme, these patients experience morbid waiting for death, believing that, for them, active living is over. There may be frequent thoughts of dying and of giving up rehabilitation efforts.

## Therapeutic Strategies

Working with aged patients can be most effective if caretakers recognize the foregoing characteristics commonly seen in older populations and design environments and treatment routines (contingencies of reinforcement) that are appropriate to the patient's level of ability and that shape his best functioning. We should keep in mind the following principles.

*Treat the Patient Respectfully.* It is essential to enhance autonomy and dignity by showing respect and concern for the individual's unique personality, preferences, and needs. Therapeutic treatments should be organized to intrude as little as possible on well-established routines and pleasures (the time the person typically rises and goes to bed or the kind of meals eaten). Also, wherever possible, the person should be given choices and opportunities for making decisions, from what to wear to informed consent regarding treatments. Even when the patient seems confused or disoriented, some simple choices can be given. His decisions, requests, and repeated statements can provide clues to significant concerns and needs that, if tended to, may improve the patient's condition or at least ease his mind.

It is wise to respect the age differences that often exist between older people and their caretakers. It is most appropriate to address patients by their last names unless invited to do otherwise and, of course, to speak to them in an adult manner, even if what is said is simplified in content and stated slowly to facilitate understanding. Balancing the direction of caring and expertise also can be particularly helpful in building rapport with an older patient. This can be accomplished, for example, by asking her about things with which she is knowledgeable, such as her profession, or allowing advice to be offered. In this manner, caretakers can acknowledge the older individual's experience in living, areas of competence, and accomplishments.

*Offer Social Support.* Most elderly patients, particularly when hospitalized and experiencing greater than normal stress, seem to crave human contact. This can be seen by the patients' often voluble conversation and obvious appreciation when someone takes time to visit and talk with them. Thus, caretakers' using time to talk with and listen to patients can be tremendously helpful in lifting their mood and maintaining their best functioning. Listening to their remembrances of past years, which is a common focus of older people's conversation, can be particularly therapeutic, as it allows patients to take pleasure in fond memories and put a lifetime of experience in some perspective. It also helps the listener to learn more about the individual patient, her past pleasures and sources of pride, her likes and dislikes, and her perceptions of her current situation. This information can be used therapeutically to arrange conditions most likely to motivate her to make her best rehabilitative efforts.

*Accommodate Degenerative Changes.* When interacting with an elderly patient, caretakers should plan their behavior and the physical environment with consideration for the person's intellectual and physical abilities (see previous discussion of degenerative changes, and Chapters 3 and 4). Avoid abrupt changes, pace conversation and activity, and allow adequate time for the person to understand and respond thoughtfully. Visual materials should be appropriate to the person's visual acuity, and spoken words or music should be loud enough for the person to hear. Glasses or hearing aids, of course, should be prescribed, if needed. When memory is a problem, it is helpful to remind the person that a particular event will be happening, especially if it is out of the ordinary or is an event for which he should have a particular mental set (see sections on memory in Chapters 4, 9, and 10). For example, reminding him that a medical test is forthcoming and that breakfast will be late, or that there will be special visitors, will help his equanimity and ability to cooperate with what will ensue. When an abrupt, possibly upsetting change will take place, it is highly desirable that a familiar person be there to remind the patient that this was an expected event and that it is for his benefit.

In accordance with patients' lowered energy and endurance, plans for care should avoid excessive fatigue. Overstimulation should be avoided, and intermittent periods of rest and relaxation should be scheduled. It is advisable to help the patient identify priorities for expending limited energy and pace herself for maximizing the amount that can be accomplished.

*Recognize Possible Neurological Pathology.*   Although certain degenerative changes can be expected in elderly populations, marked psychological deficits, and certainly any abrupt change in functioning, should be examined closely. Consultation with neurologists, psychiatrists, and psychologists would be most appropriate in identifying neurological pathology (tumor, dementia) and in discriminating these from psychological disorders (pseudodementia, depression).

*Recognize and Treat Depression.*   Be alert to evidence of depression, which may be related to too few pleasurable activities, placement with patients who are either much more or much less deteriorated, loss of autonomy, loneliness, loss of hope, or thoughts of death. Diversion and involvement in activities are important therapeutic strategies for minimizing depression, isolation, and lack of intellectual stimulation, all of which are particularly common during hospitalization. One of the best means of increasing involvement is to encourage patients to mingle in a common room, play cards or engage in other social activities, and share mealtimes. This encourages mutual emotional support among patients, as well as some intellectual challenge, and provides an environment that approaches the kind of social belonging that probably characterized the individual's world during "healthy" periods.

It also is important to look for incentives that would be particularly meaningful. These incentives then can be used to reward activities considered beneficial for the patient (therapy, grooming). For example, a patient may be given a pass for lunch with a friend (if this pleases her) following her demonstration that she can walk independently to the end of the hall. Such contingencies can be structured by the staff as natural consequences of progress, or they may be agreed upon by both the staff and patient as a means of generating personal goals and stimulating greater incentive for the patient's own efforts.

Discussion of depressive thoughts, particularly of losses and death, should be engaged in if the patient initiates or communicates a need to talk of these thoughts. In excess, however, discussion and continued focus on death or the frustrations of old age may become counterproductive and serve to reinforce the patient's negative thoughts and mood. It is helpful, therefore, as a general rule, to keep discussions cheerful and centered about pleasant topics, remembrances, or future prospects (perhaps of the visits of children and grandchildren). Such positive conversation typically lifts the patient's mood, at least temporarily, and interrupts ruminative negative thoughts. The more serious discussion of fears, worries, and concerns is best left to occur at specified times between the patient and a few intimate others or a mental-health professional.

*Maximize Familiarity and Organization in the Environment.* To enhance a sense of security, increase the likelihood of effective coping, and facilitate orientation for the confused, patients should remain in familiar surroundings, insofar as possible. When hospitalized, it is helpful for the patient to stay in the same room and have some familiar articles in his possession, such as his own robe and slippers, family pictures, and radio. For example, one elderly man was greatly comforted by the presence of his own chest of drawers and an old, particularly prized family clock. Continuity of schedule and personnel and the presence of orienting materials such as clocks, calendars, and windows also may help the elderly avoid excessive anxiety, disorientation, and confusion (see Chapters 4 and 10).

*Organize Community Resources.* For an elderly, disabled person, social isolation and the threat of not being able to maintain independent living are persistent problems. Home assistance programs, such as those available through the Visiting Nurses Association and Meals on Wheels (see Appendix E), can provide personal and homemaking aid. Older people should be encouraged to seek social activities by participating, for example, in community-interest groups (book clubs, civic organizations) and senior citizens' centers. They also may find it beneficial to contact the Grey Panthers and the American Association for Retired Persons, which are concerned specifically with rights, opportunities, and resources for older individuals.

# 12    The Patient Who Is Young

## Children and Young Adults

For our purposes, *pediatric patient* will refer to any patient under the age of 16 and *young adult patient* will refer to those between the ages of 16 and approximately 30. These patients may be grouped together because, despite differences, they share several important characteristics associated with youth and their stages of development. For example, the pediatric patient usually lives in a nuclear family, is dependent upon parents or legal guardians, and has yet to establish an independent lifestyle, an enduring intimate relationship, or a vocational commitment. Also, although many individuals between the ages of 20 and 30 have made social and vocational commitments, many have not, and all must be considered relatively new to the responsibilities of adulthood. Along with the pediatric patient, they "have their futures before them." Additionally, because of the young body's good recuperative powers, children and young adults often have the best prognoses for dramatic and sustained recovery after injury. Thus, rehabilitation with this population holds an excellent potential to enhance significantly patients' health, achievements, and life satisfactions.

### Areas of Disrupted Functioning

Accidental injury is the most frequent cause of disability among pediatric and young-adult patients. Broken bones, burns, and head or spinal-cord injuries are the most common. Chronic diseases, such as leukemia, juvenile diabetes, rheumatoid arthritis, renal failure, and multiple sclerosis also may result in the need for rehabilitation services. These disparate conditions, of course, result in varying kinds and degrees of cognitive and emotional changes. General strategies for understanding and treating a range of these problems (neurological deficit, depression, anxiety) can be found in this book's earlier chapters; however, several other areas of functioning that are particularly important with young populations and may be disrupted by disability will be discussed in the next few sections.

*Parent-Child Relations.*   Nearly all pediatric and young adult patients depend upon their parents or legal guardians for support and care to a later age than do healthy peers. The child who has been chronically ill or disabled tends to live at home longer than does a healthy child; and the young adult who has lived independently and then becomes disabled often returns at least temporarily to the parental household. Young married patients frequently separate and "go home," despite genuine caring between the spouses, when the relatively new relationship cannot accommodate the changes imposed by disability. The young patient's need for daily assistance (in personal care, mobility), his limited financial resources, and his psychological status combine to prolong his dependence upon parents.

When a young person's life revolves around parents for a long period of time, problems often arise with regard to parental overprotection and the child's overdependency. Parents may establish excessive control and do too much for their child in areas where she could manage successfully on her own, such as household chores, arranging services in the community, and getting around the neighborhood. It is not uncommon for parents to baby their "sick" child and fail to respect her age and retained competencies; consequently, she may have difficulty in establishing independent activities and associations and in making independent decisions.

An example is provided by a 25-year-old man who suffered a spinal-cord injury, prior to which he had worked full time, lived independently, and had been engaged to be married. Immediately following his injury, he found his hospital room overflowing with stuffed animals and childish trinkets sent by his parents, who spoke to him in a condescending manner, tried to anticipate and satisfy all of his needs, and required little of him in terms of initiation or assertion. This babying and protective manner, although initially comforting to the patient, soon became problematic; the man's dependent attitude and powerless status as a patient was emphasized, and his passive role in rehabilitation was reinforced. It became difficult for therapists to communicate with him directly, and he appeared increasingly depressed as he exerted decreasing control over his environment and engaged in fewer activities on his own initiative.

For the young child, in particular, overprotection and babying may be associated with inadequate discipline. Some parents, who see their child as disadvantaged due to disability, shy away from setting firm limits and following through with discipline. They often report feeling that disciplining a "sick" child is overly harsh, and they act as if their leniency could make up for the disadvantages and distress the child suffers. Such a parenting approach may well lead to behavior problems that have far-reaching, disruptive effects upon the child's relationship with peers, figures of authority (teachers and, later, bosses), and family members.

For example, the parents of an eight-year-old boy with rheumatoid arthritis imposed very few demands upon him and tried to satisfy all his desires, often at the expense of their own needs. They did not expect him to contribute to the household by doing chores, and they consistently did much for him that he could have done for himself, such as getting himself to school and making his own snacks. As a result, the boy's dependent and demanding behaviors were reinforced and became increasingly troublesome. He became tyrannical at home, demanding service and excessive attention, and failed to develop skills either for cooperating with others or for functioning effectively on his own.

At an extreme, inadequate discipline and parental overprotection or domination disrupt the developmental progress typically associated with the child's age. For example, a toddler's direct knowledge of the world, tolerance for frustration, and ability to master new materials and situations can be diminished when others consistently anticipate and satisfy her needs, instruct her in how to solve novel problems, make few demands upon her to master appropriately graded tasks, and restrict her movement and ventures of discovery. Similarly, an adolescent's establishment of healthy, same-sex and heterosexual relationships can be forestalled when family members discourage increasing independence, peer-oriented cooperation, and self-confidence, and instead reward him for depending upon and staying close to family members and expressing ideas in complete accord with their own.

*Social Relationships beyond the Family.* Disability that distinguishes a patient from most other people typically results in some degree of social isolation and alienation. Isolation results from both environmental and psychological conditions. For example, practical environmental or medical considerations frequently exclude, at least for some time, the young patient from school, recreational ventures, jobs, or community activities that make up the normal social world. For the pediatric patient in particular, early exclusion from the peer milieu may obstruct development of age-appropriate social skills and peer (as opposed to adult) orientation.

In addition to these practical barriers, the young disabled person often is psychologically isolated by feelings of being "different" or "abnormal." Social sensitivity and feelings of rejection, of course, are exacerbated easily by the experience of being a target of ridicule or public curiosity. Such feelings result in increasing social anxiety, which in turn leads to the person's further isolation and avoidance of social situations. Accumulated feelings of social inadequacy and isolation lead many disabled young people simply to assume they will not achieve the social life that they desire and feel is possible for others; thus, they experience persistent depression and loneliness. Such individuals become increasingly delayed in the acquisition of social skills and self-confidence.

As an illustration, we may consider the 25-year-old woman with kidney disease who had been on dialysis since mid-adolescence. She described herself as shy, particularly with men, and uncomfortable concerning others' reactions to her condition. She was uncertain when to tell new acquaintances about her illness, and expected people to shy away from her after learning of her disease and her need for continuing dialysis. Moreover, since much of her time and energy had to be expended in the treatment of her illness, she lacked a variety of experiences that young people often share and can talk about, such as skiing, traveling, and working. She also lacked dating experience, which, as she got older, became more and more a barrier between herself and men, and even a barrier between herself and women friends who had had greater experience. As a result of her anxieties and lack of skill, she avoided social situations, despite loneliness and a genuine desire for companionship. In so doing, she suffered escalating feelings of social inadequacy and depression.

Social anxiety and alienation can be particularly great when a person's disability involves sexual dysfunction (spinal-cord injury) or body disfigurement (burns or amputation). If the person feels unattractive and sexually inadequate, many hopes held prior to disability or held by healthy peers, such as hopes for love, marriage, parenthood, and community acceptance, are abandoned. Such a person often narrows his range of activity and social interactions and thereby limits his access to a wide range of reinforcements. This social isolation and limited reinforcement, in turn, exacerbate feelings of depression and of course do nothing to develop the person's positive social skills or prove to himself that he might, in fact, enjoy and succeed in activities he currently avoids. The brain-injured patient (see Chapter 9) is particularly likely to suffer social isolation, as she may have difficulty in getting around, communicating with others, and, most importantly, maintaining appropriate self-control and behaving in accordance with social norms. In most communities there are few social activities in which brain-injured people can participate, thus adding to their social problems.

*Educational, Vocational, and Recreational Opportunities.* Regardless of an individual's level of functioning, the establishment of patterns for learning, working, and enjoying recreation is essential for achieving structure, stimulation, and meaning in life. To the extent that patients fail to establish goals, patterns of interest, and skills, they are apt to feel bored, unproductive, and inadequate, and suffer consequent dissatisfaction.

Educational adjustment is a central concern in the lives of children, and vocational satisfaction is a critical aspect in the lives of young adults. Therefore, pediatric patients are particularly vulnerable to learning difficulties, while young adults are most vulnerable to poor vocational adjustment. Of course, the likelihood of one's gaining access to and succeeding in an educational or vocational program is determined by the nature and extent of the person's disability. Clearly, a paraplegic cannot be a construction worker, and a child with significant brain damage cannot participate in regular academic programs or be groomed for a college education. In addition to limitations in functioning, such practical problems as finances and transportation, such social barriers as others' lack of information and their intolerance, and psychological problems in attitudinal, social, and emotional adjustment all add to the challenge of educational and vocational rehabilitation.

## Therapeutic Strategies

As we have emphasized repeatedly, treatment strategies need to be tailored to the individual patient's circumstances, beliefs, and feelings concerning herself and her world, as well as the observable conditions of reinforcement that influence her thoughts and behaviors. General approaches to working with pediatric and young-adult patients can be formulated, however, with an eye to the social, familial, vocational, and educational difficulties to which this population is particularly vulnerable. These are as follows.

*Teach and Reward Age-Appropriate Behavior.* Caretakers should arrange the patient's environment to shape and reward her doing independently as much as possible and her mastering increasingly complex and novel tasks and situations. It is important not to anticipate and satisfy all of a patient's needs or restrict her direct experience of the environment. Instead, allow her to recognize needs (know what she wants), develop skills to satisfy them (gain reinforcement), and take reasonable risks in new circumstances (rather than avoid them) without excessive fear.

Expectations for the patient need to be appropriate for her age and psychological functioning. Whatever her level, however, she should be given responsibility for some tasks upon which reinforcement (some pleasure or privilege) is contingent. For the toddler, responsibilities might be that of complying with adult directions, while for the older child it could be taking care of personal hygiene and some household chores. For the young adult, it might consist of seeking employment.

Rewards and social encouragement for increasingly independent and responsible behaviors must be appropriate to the patient's age and cognitive ability. For example, stars and colorful stickers for desirable behaviors may be rewarding for a youngster but insulting to an adolescent. Similarly, praise and feedback must not sound condescending and should not smack of babying, in either tone of voice or content, for adolescent and adult patients. Attention and discussions usually are rewarding at any age, as is sharing an activity in one of the patient's chosen areas of interest.

*Support Social Activities with Peers.* A young patient's interactions with family and caretakers must be complemented by peer-oriented social activities. Because chronically disabled young patients may be excluded from normal socialization, it is important to arrange involvement in peer groups so that they can learn appropriate social behavior and may experience the rewards of friendship (fun, knowledge, support). Young, intellectually impaired patients, in particular, will benefit from structured social activities, and, at times, direct training to help them learn or relearn appropriate social behavior (see Chapter 9).

During hospitalization, a patient is likely to benefit from rooming with patients who are perceived as similar, perhaps in age, interests, or life circumstances. A playroom for young children, the canteen, or a dining room can provide a setting for social interactions and activity. In the community, a person's participation in recreational activities, classes, or volunteer work, will increase opportunities to develop friendships and a sense of social belonging. The societies designed to assist people with particular disabilites (Multiple Sclerosis Society, Cancer Foundation) also sponsor activities designed to promote social support and recreation. In addition, at some point, even the young adult who cannot live independently might benefit from leaving the parental home and living with adequate assistance elsewhere (a group home or a room-and-board establishment), preferably with other young people.

*Initiate Counseling with the Patient.* As with people of any age, pediatric and young-adult patients should receive psychological treatment as soon as emotional or behavioral disturbances are identified. In addition, because of this population's high risk for life disruptions associated with disability, intervention frequently is advisable as a preventive strategy.

Counseling with the patient typically involves a combination of listening, to identify and clarify the patient's thoughts and feelings; offering information, at a level understandable to the patient; and guiding problem solving. Counseling should help the person to recognize and modify maladaptive behaviors and attitudes, identify and maximize strengths and assets, and cope realistically with circumstances that will not change. It is particularly important to talk with adolescents and young adults about social relations and sexual behavior. A young person with a disabling condition, like any other young person, needs to learn social skills that will maintain positive interpersonal relationships, as well as when and how sexual activity can become an appropriate part of a relationship. For example, patients with spinal-cord injuries need information on their sexual potential and options and often need support and guidance in handling their new sexual roles within the nondisabled social milieu. Similarly, the young brain-injured patient may need to learn (or relearn) the sexual facts, in terms comprehensible to him, and how to discriminate appropriate versus inappropriate social behavior.

The effectiveness of direct counseling with adolescents and adults depends, to a great extent, upon the patient's cognitive ability to examine conditions influencing his behavior, including private, social, and environmental factors. He then must be able to arrange these influences to support or reinforce healthy, adjustive behaviors and to discourage or extinguish less desirable behaviors. Young children and patients with significant intellectual deficits, therefore, are not well suited to a psychotherapeutic approach. Although they may benefit from the supportive or directly educational nature of counseling, their optimal adjustment is most likely to be accomplished by structuring the external environment so that it shapes their best adjustment. In these cases, the key to success lies in teaching patients' family members and caretakers how to interact therapeutically with them and how to structure naturally therapeutic environments.

*Initiate Family Counseling.*   This is essential with families of chronically ill or disabled children and may range from continuing discussion of the child's medical condition, developmental progress, and psychological adjustment, to guidance with particular problems. Such problems may be the child's fearfulness, depression, or behavioral disruption or the family's lack of discipline, their own depression, or their feelings of guilt. Counseling should focus both on the family's adjustment to their child's difficulties (see Chapter 13) and on teaching them to interact with the child to facilitate her greatest adjustment and rehabilitation. For example, parents might be taught communication skills (praising, active listening) and behavioral methods of discipline (rewarding, "time-out" procedures for noncompliance) in order to modify a child's disruptive behavior. [See, for example, Becker's *Parents are Teachers* (1971) and Patterson and Gullion's *Living with Children* (1968).] In counseling, parents often are asked to assume the role of therapist as well as that of parent. Within this framework, parents must learn to become astute observers and managers of behavior (see Chapter 3).

The participation of parents and, when available, the patient's partner (spouse, girlfriend, or boyfriend) is critical in rehabilitation of the young-adult patient. Counseling with parents often focuses on the necessity of their resuming parenting responsibilities for their offspring, who is now an adult. With the spouse, counseling centers on private feelings and concerns, observable ways in which the couple interact, and practical options (financial, vocational, sexual) for patient and spouse. When an individual's disability occurs after the couple's initial commitment, the spouse's possible ambivalence for continued commitment should be explored. This may be a particularly difficult and complex issue when the patient's disability involves neuropsychological impairment, sexual dysfunction, disfigurement, or significant motoric limitations.

Further discussion of family adjustment will be presented in Chapter 13.

*Provide Educational Consultation.*   Federal law mandates that special educational services be provided for all handicapped children until the age of 21. "Handicapped" includes those children with specific learning disabilities, intellectual deficits, physical disabilities, or emotional/behavioral disturbances. Schools must teach skills appropriate to the individual's level of functioning and use educational techniques most likely to facilitate that person's learning. The academic setting must be as nearly "normal" (as minimally restrictive) as possible. School options such as home instruction, small-group tutoring, special classroom instruction, and alternative, nonacademic, programming can be considered. If the child's neighborhood school cannot meet his needs, placement elsewhere must be arranged at the school's expense.

As soon as a school-aged child is recognized as limited in his ability to participate or learn in a regular classroom, the child's school should be notified. Occasionally, of course, the school itself recognizes the problem first and contacts the parents. In either case, school officials, with the parents' consent, gather evaluation data. After obtaining assessments from appropriate sources (teacher, physician, psychologist, educational specialist), an Individualized Education Program (IEP) is established, again with parents' consent. The IEP describes the child's level of functioning, the proposed educational goals (one year at a time), and the strategies that will be used to attain the goals.

Learning specialists and psychologists typically have central roles in assessing a child's educational needs and recommending courses of action to school faculties. Speech pathologists, physical and occupational therapists, and physicians also should make assessments and recommendations specific to language, physical, or medical problems. For example, if a child has an aphasic language disorder following a head injury, he needs an educational program designed in consultation with a speech pathologist. Without this language expertise, teachers might offer the child individual and extra attention, or they might treat him as if he were a slow learner but continue to use regular teaching techniques. They might not recognize that his special needs were circumscribed and that he had important areas of maintained competence.

As demonstrated in this example, children with neurological impairments are probably those most in need of expert consultation in educational planning. School faculties typically lack experience with this population and cannot assess readily the complex factors influencing the child's behavior. In addition, individual behavior problems, particularly of a social nature, often are manifested by these children, and guidance regarding behavioral management is essential. In this case, a professional would assist teachers and school staff to understand the child's behavior and to establish a program designed to achieve behavioral control at school.

*Initiate Vocational Rehabilitation.* Vocational training and rehabilitation are designed to guide an individual into some form of productive work appropriate to her level of functioning, considering all of her strengths, weaknesses, and interests. For an individual who had established a career that could not be continued following disability, retraining in a new field would be needed. For the individual who had not yet established career goals, initial evaluation and training would be appropriate.

Vocational plans should be based upon comprehensive assessment of the individual's intellectual abilities, specific talents, physical functioning (skill, endurance), social skills, and behavioral characteristics (tolerance of frustration, distractability, emotional control). Individual interests, likes and dislikes, and general attitudes and values also must be considered. Such assessments typically are accomplished by psychologists, vocational counselors, and, when appropriate, other professionals who are involved in the particular person's care.

People over 21 years of age, or several years younger if no longer associated with the public schools (or if referred by them), may take advantage of services offered by the Vocational Rehabilitation Department. This state agency secures assessments for clients and offers vocational counseling and planning. Once a plan is established, funds typically are provided to support the individual's training, which may involve a return to school or direct placement for on-the-job experience. Homebound work, and part-time positions also may be considered. The Vocational Rehabilitation Department can provide a client with appropriate transportation (hand controls for a paraplegic's car) or other special equipment (typewriter, electronic communicator) that would promote his work potential and performance. If a person's skills are inadequate for competitive employment, she may be placed appropriately at a sheltered workshop, where she will receive close supervision. Although this chapter focuses on relatively young patients, vocational rehabilitation, of course, can be appropriate for any disabled adult interested in developing work skills.

Occasionally, a person will "fall through the cracks" of a large agency such as the Vocational Rehabilitation Department. Patients, family members, and rehabilitation workers should be vigilant to see that this does not occur. Rehabilitation therapists, in particular, can be invaluable as patient advocates, to assure timely referral and appropriate follow-through for vocational training.

# IV

# Coping Skills for Caretakers

# 13    Family Adjustment

Disability affects not only patients but also those with whom their lives are intimately connected; most notably, spouses and other family members. These individuals, as well as the patient, experience considerable change and stress as a result of the patient's impaired functioning, and they need time and assistance in order to adjust. Unfortunately, rehabilitation services, and families themselves, often emphasize care of the patient while giving too little attention to changes occurring within the family. It typically is discovered, however, that the family's adjustment and the patient's rehabilitation are intertwined inextricably and that one is neglected only with great detriment to the other. For example, it would be hard to imagine a patient's adjusting well to a medical crisis or chronic disability in the midst of a distraught and stressful home environment. On the other hand, the patient with an emotionally supportive family that understands her difficulties and encourages rehabilitative efforts is likely to do as well as possible. Of course, in addition to facilitating the patient's progress, it is in itself a valued goal to help family members feel better and cope more effectively with the patient. Thus, although the primary focus of a rehabilitation program is the patient, the concerns and needs of significant others must be considered.

## Conditions Contributing to a Family's Emotional Stress

During crises, family members frequently show symptoms of moderate to severe stress and associated symptoms of depression and anxiety, such as difficulty in concentrating, sleep disturbance, increased somatic complaints, distractibility, increased emotionality, or decreased efficiency at work (see Chapters 5 and 6). This stress results from the tremendous life changes associated with one member's disability, as well as from feelings of sadness and frustration in response to a loved one's unfortunate condition. Family disruption often is particularly great (1) when a patient's disabling condition is of sudden onset, as with injuries following an accident; (2) during initial diagnosis of any condition; and (3) when the cumulative effects of a progressive illness result in a precipitous decline in functioning. Although examination of particular circumstances is the best means of identifying the stressors affecting a given family, the following conditions impinge on almost all families and contribute significantly to their emotional upheaval.

*Empathy for the Patient.*   It is painful to see a loved one severely ill or incapacitated for what may be a prolonged period of time. The patient's pain, suffering, and discouragement easily can pervade the entire family atmosphere because all empathize and "feel for" him. The former athlete may be confined to a wheelchair, a competent business manager may be unable to trust his own computations and judgments, and a loving mother may be unable to speak intelligibly to her children. Family members share feelings of sadness and loss in these circumstances, and at times they can be overwhelmed with the recognition of how much less able the patient is than she was when healthy, or could have been expected to be under other circumstances.

*Role Changes.*   As mentioned in Chapter 1, when a family member cannot continue to assume his usual roles and responsibilities, relationships within the family necessarily change. For example, the patient no longer may be able to be the breadwinner for the family, the responsible parent for the children, or the one who keeps the checking account straight, fixes the car, or cooks the meals. Previously equal and sharing relationships, such as that between spouses, may become unequal as the healthy partner assumes most of the family responsibilities. By the same token, previously unequal relationships, such as that between a parent and a child, may become reversed so that the child cares for the parent. Since an individual's feeling of identity is determined largely by his activities and relationships with significant others, such major changes in roles and in established balances of power produce dramatic disruption in how both patient and family members see themselves. In fact, patients and family members often describe feelings of depersonalization in that they simply do not recognize themselves in the lives they now lead.

*Assumption of Additional Responsibilities.*   As stated previously, family members often are required to assume new responsibilities, learn new behaviors, and fill roles previously assumed by the patient, in addition to maintaining most of their usual responsibilities. For example, a woman who never worked outside the home during her marriage may need to seek vocational training if her husband is unable to work. At the same time, she must continue to shoulder most of her usual homemaking responsibilities and, in addition, will need to make arrangements for the care of her spouse.

Similarly, a man may need to learn how to balance the checkbook, do the grocery shopping, and find more time to spend with the children, as well as visit his wife at the hospital or transport her for treatments. When a parent is disabled, children may have to be more subdued, take over some home chores, assume independent care of themselves after school, or even help care for the patient.

*Loss of Independence.* Typically, when family members assume new responsibilities to meet the demands of the situation, they pay dearly in terms of time, energy, and freedom. As more demands are placed upon them, they find less time to pursue their usual, preferred activities and have fewer opportunities to attend to their own personal needs. For example, many family members must curtail social and recreational activities severely during the patient's rehabilitation period; only perceived necessities are accomplished, and most efforts at enjoyment or relaxation are forgone. The loss of pleasurable activities and of perceived freedom, added to the rigorous schedule of often minimally rewarding responsibilities, contributes significantly to family members' weariness, irritability, depression, and, at times, resentment.

*Loss of Support, Affection, and Security.* When confronted with catastrophic injury, patients often are unable to continue to meet the emotional needs of others; thus, their families lose this important source of emotional support. Many patients become self-centered as a result of their own distress, and some (especially those with brain injury) lose the social sensitivity and awareness that normally would enable them to respond appropriately to family members' feelings. The patient's self-centeredness or social insensitivity may be transient or may persist for quite some time.

Changes in sexual feelings and behavior may give rise to particular stress and loss of support between spouses. Although decline of sexual interest is common during periods of stress (and, for the patient, physical compromise), the spouse of such a disinterested individual may find it hard to tolerate abstinence over an extended period of time. Feelings of loneliness and rejection may result. Moreover, for many reasons, a healthy spouse may discourage sexual advances from the patient. For example, she may fear hurting the patient, or she may have altered feelings resulting from the patient's decreased capabilities or changed appearance. The patient in such a case is likely to feel extremely sensitive to perceived rejection because, as a result of his disability or disfigurement, he may see himself as sexually unattractive or even repugnant. Even the healthy spouse who initiates the sexual separation suffers from sexual frustration, loss of affection, and loneliness. Feelings of guilt for having rejected the partner are likely to add to distress. As described in Chapter 12, poor social and sexual adjustment typically are greatest for patients with neurological deficits, impaired sexual functioning, or significant disfigurement.

Decreased feelings of security and stability affect all family members who have depended upon the patient for functions she no longer is able to perform. Financial insecurity and loss of social status frequently are experienced when the primary worker in the family is disabled and unemployed. Similarly, children with a newly disabled parent are likely to be stressed by the loss of the parent's emotionally stabilizing influence, authority, and judgment. The children may miss the parent as participant and teacher in many activities; the losses, of course, depend upon the areas of deficit suffered by the patient.

*Fear of the Future.*   For caring family members and significant others, the uncertainty of their loved one's prognosis is a continual source of frustration and anxiety. The family must hold future plans and permanent decisions in abeyance until it can be determined what level of functioning the patient will attain. The problems that will have to be faced, therefore, remain unclear and are not immediately soluble, leaving fertile ground for ruminative worry and fearfulness.

## Helping Families to Cope

As indicated earlier in this chapter, family members' emotional adjustment is important both for the family's own sake and for the patient's. It cannot be overstated that a patient's rehabilitation is influenced heavily by the stability and security she senses within the family. Attitudes and behaviors such as acceptance, helpfulness, respect, and patience in allowing the patient to progress at her own pace provide the conditions for the best learning, motivation, and emotional stability. Alternatively, the family's nonacceptance, disrespect, intolerance, and associated punitive behaviors often result in poor progress, lack of motivation, and emotional instability. Therefore, even though troublesome emotional reactions within the family may be normal and expected during rehabilitation, they should not be accepted or ignored; rather, family members should be helped to analyze their feelings and behavior, plan self-help strategies, and seek psychological treatment when negative emotions and behaviors interfere with their daily functioning or their ability to interact therapeutically with the patient. Although coping strategies for family members will depend upon the particular needs and resources of the individuals involved, the following general suggestions should be considered.

*Keep the Family Informed.*   Families should be given full and clear information concerning the patient's medical and psychological status and what might be anticipated. This information can help families to make sense of the patient's otherwise often incomprehensible behavior, to avoid becoming unduly upset, and, thus, to respond to the patient most therapeutically. For example, if family members know that the patient's severe anxiety is a causal factor in his complaining, negativistic, and at times explosive and accusatory behavior, they are less likely to respond angrily or to personalize insults. Instead, they may be able to remain more objective, plan their responses to decrease the patient's anxiety, and avoid exciting or reinforcing his continued undesirable behaviors (see Chapter 3).

*Encourage Family Members to Express Thoughts and Feelings.* As discussed in earlier chapters, sharing concerns often makes them easier to bear. When personal thoughts are spoken aloud, the speaker often for the first time recognizes particularly disturbing aspects of the situation. This identification of problems, of course, is prerequisite to developing effective solutions. In addition to improving personal problem solving, discussion invites others to share viewpoints and suggestions that may prove useful. Moreover, sharing thoughts and feelings typically results in an individual's feeling understood, supported, and not alone. Under such conditions, people usually report feeling better and can be observed to function more effectively.

*Prompt Families to Seek Help from Others.* One cannot be expected to handle everything independently under the best of circumstances, and certainly not at times of family crisis when responsibilities are greatly increased and stress reduces the individual's capacity for concentration and patience. Support from extended family and friends is absolutely necessary at this time, and their offers of help should not be rejected for fear of inconveniencing them. Often, professionals, friends, or community agencies already have accumulated relevant information that they would be pleased to share. Family members also might benefit from being introduced to the families of other patients with whom they can share experiences, information, and support.

Help also should be sought from friends, family members, or professionals, when the patient needs significant assistance or supervision at home. One family member's attempt to do it all is unreasonable, if not impossible, and often contributes to role strains in the family. For example, relentlessly unequal patient/caretaker roles can be disruptive for a married couple or for a parent and child who previously interacted in reversed power roles. In this case, outside care should be encouraged in order to avoid conflicts between patient and family and to avoid interference with what the family can provide best, namely, love, caring, and emotional support. For example, it may be preferable for an employed caretaker, rather than a spouse, to clean bowel accidents if they occur. Otherwise, this unpleasant occurrence may affect adversely the feelings of affection, respect, dignity, and sexual interest between patient and spouse. These affectional bonds are difficult for the spouse to maintain through repeated, unrelieved experience as nurse, housemaid, or babysitter, and they are far too precious to place in jeopardy. Employed help is not only a boon to the family; the patient also probably will benefit from contact with people outside the family.

*Advise and Reward Families' Being Good to Themselves.*  Families should be helped to recognize that, during this stressful time, it is important that they be good to their bodies and attentive to their own emotional needs. It is important to get sufficient rest, eat properly, maintain contact with friends, and keep some time just for personal concerns. Nonessential chores can be discarded temporarily, and involvement in some assumed responsibilities (participation in community services) might be eased.

Nobody can or should try to spend all of his time and energy with, or thinking about, the patient. Time and thought elsewhere provide diversion and stimulation that can improve spirits and revitalize the individual for more hard work with the patient. Outside interests also enable the family member to bring home news or new thoughts to share with the patient, thereby expanding her interests, improving her morale, and increasing her motivation to return to a more active life. Thus, family members should plan to get out of the house or away from the hospital occasionally, see friends, and continue participation in at least some activities of interest (hobbies, sports, clubs, work). The patient also typically feels good about family members' maintaining these activities, because it relieves guilt about "trapping" or burdening them.

*Suggest Relaxation.*  Family members, like patients, benefit from engaging in relaxing activities (hiking, listening to music, cooking), or from practicing specific relaxation techniques, such as that detailed in Appendix D. Relaxation helps relieve tension and feelings of anxiety and can be a welcome "time out" from problems and a busy schedule.

*Shape Family Members' Personal Coping and Skill with the Patient.*  As it has been stressed throughout this book regarding patients, families too can become more effective if professionals and others will give effort to shaping their behavior. Thus, we must not expect families to adjust to changes and learn to care for the patient quickly or entirely at one time; rather, adjustment and skilled care will develop in a step-wise fashion of increasingly more effective behavior. In light of this, rehabilitation workers must set appropriate expectations for family members and assure that reinforcement is adequate to keep families trying and feeling reasonably optimistic. At first, families should be praised for doing what they can manage easily, for example, visiting the patient in the hospital regularly. Next, they might be encouraged and complimented for attending therapies with the patient; then, for asking appropriate questions; then, for proposing alternative solutions to questions raised; then, for increasing involvement in the patient's direct care. As described in Chapter 3, we must arrange conditions to make it most likely that families will behave effectively, and then we must reward appropriate behavior, pay little attention to or supportively correct less appropriate behavior, and avoid criticism. Direct criticism or confrontation, regarding, for example, the family's less-than-optimal cooperation or therapeutic behavior with the patient, is unlikely to produce positive change. It is more likely that the family will withdraw from professionals who criticize and will ignore or oppose their information and advice. Unfortunately, this in turn frequently results in serious problems for the patient.

*Encourage Family Counseling.* Rehabilitation often is a long, slow process that can, without expert guidance, involve severe family strains detrimental to all involved. It therefore frequently is advisable for family members, particularly a spouse, the parents of disabled children, or the primary caretaker, to talk with a mental-health professional who is knowledgeable about rehabilitation. The patient may or may not be present during these discussions, depending on his condition and the content of the talk. Professional consultation from time to time can help to identify specific problems and encourage consideration of alternative solutions before the problems become chronic. By talking with a counselor about conflicting emotions and difficulties with the patient, family members can learn to work and live with more equanimity, stability in method and purpose, and greater reward.

# 14 Stress Management for the Professional

Working with medically ill or physically disabled people, although rewarding in many ways, is a stressful and psychologically demanding task. It is important for the professional (physician, nurse, therapist, aide, home helper) to be aware that work-related stress is experienced by nearly everyone and can be predicted to affect personal functioning and work efficiency. Such awareness should prompt the professional to be vigilant for signs of stress in her own and her colleagues' behavior. She then can attempt conscientiously to reorganize conditions at work and elsewhere so that they stimulate and reward better adjustment. Of course, optimal patient care also is more likely to come from psychologically healthy caretakers who are not experiencing undue stress. Therefore, successful stress reduction programs should result in both an improved quality of life for the professional and better care for the patient.

## Signs of Stress

Work-related stress can affect professionals in a variety of ways, depending upon the individual's personality, his characteristic style of coping, and his personal resources outside of work. Common signs of stress are depression (see Chapter 5), anxiety (see Chapter 6), easy fatigue, physical illness (indigestion, tension headaches), loss of emotional control (quickness to anger, oversensitivity), and loss of efficiency and flexibility in thinking. For example, a nurse may find herself snapping at patients or begrudgingly and slowly answering calls for assistance. Similarly, a therapist may be annoyed by a patient's anxiety and hesitancy in trying a new activity, or by a colleague's request for assistance. A physician may be curt with nurses or repeatedly unavailable to patients. Most professionals probably recall mornings when getting out of bed was a major effort and having to respond to patients' needs felt nearly impossible because of personal concerns and emotions. The detrimental consequences of stress at work can spread beyond the work environment and affect the individual's family life, social relationships, and recreational interests. These stress reactions may be acute and arise irregularly when conditions at the job are particularly demanding, or they may be chronic and result in "burnout" when excessive demands and stress persist over an extended period of time.

## Typical Stress-Inducing Situations

The conditions associated with stress-related feelings and behavior vary among people and demand individual analyses (see Chapter 3). For example, caring for patients with certain diseases or with certain personality styles may be particularly difficult for one nurse, but not for another. Such idiosyncratic reactions may be related to the nurse's own fears, personal experience with that particular disease, or past experiences of success or failure (history of reinforcement) in coping with people who have behaved similarly. The following general aspects of rehabilitation, however, often contribute significantly to the stress experienced by health-care professionals.

*Seeing Another Person's Distress.* Empathic feelings of sadness and distress typically are stimulated by observing a patient's physical pain, emotional upheaval, or declining functioning. Feelings of frustration and helplessness can result from one's own impotence to alter significantly the patient's condition. These feelings are particularly strong when a caretaker has worked with the patient over an extended period of time, identifies with him in some way (is of similar age or shares interests), or has built a candid and close relationship with him. Moreover, it is especially heartrending to see a patient face catastrophic disability with little support from family or friends. When a patient's family seems inattentive or unfeeling, empathy for the patient and hostility toward the family can be particularly great.

*Recognizing Limited Community Options.* Staff members often experience empathic distress and frustration when confronted with the "injustices" that befall patients. It is upsetting, for example, to find it necessary to arrange extended care for a patient when care at the available facility is known to be less than desirable. Similarly, it is distressing to see patients who are struggling to cope with disabilities meet discrimination and intolerance in their communities or in the marketplace. Too often, none of the rehabilitation patient's alternatives promise a desirable solution to problems, particularly when considered in relation to what could have been for that individual if he were functioning fully.

*Slow Rehabilitation Progress*.   The slowness of a patient's recovery is stressful for the therapist as well as for the patient. Because the patient's progress is a substantial part of the caretaker's professional reward (reinforcement), continued lack of, or slow, progress can have an adverse effect upon the caretaker's mood. In such circumstances, the professional at times wonders if he is doing all he can, or even if he is competent. Such self-doubts, of course, exaggerate feelings of helplessness and low self-esteem.

*Little Appreciation from Patients*.   When patients are ill and trying to cope with their own difficulties, they often are "self-centered" in the sense that they are acutely aware of their own needs and can attend little to the needs of others. This often results in many demands from patients but few thanks, smiles, or expressions of interest in the caretaker beyond her professional role. Although professionals know that they should not rely on approval and personal affirmation from patients, a relative absence of social rewards is certain to take its emotional toll on the caretaker. The more debilitated or poorly adjusted the patient, the less likely he is to behave in a socially reinforcing manner.

*Worry About One's Own Vulnerability*.   Most health-care professionals, at one time or another, confront such questions as, "What if I severed my spinal cord in an accident?" "What if I had a brain tumor?" "What if my spouse became severely impaired intellectually or physically?" or "What if my child had neurological deficits?" Although these questions may stimulate philosophically enriching speculations, they also can give rise to persistent worry or overfearfulness for oneself and overprotectiveness of loved ones. Unfortunately, anticipation of injury or disease does little to lessen the likelihood of such a medical crisis and does much to increase anxiety and stress.

## Strategies for Reducing Stress

The following suggestions can help health-care professionals to cope with the daily stress of their work. The goal of these coping strategies is not to make work with patients free of stress—that simply will not happen—but rather to moderate stress and assure that it does not result in generalized personal dissatisfaction (depression) or loss of professional effectiveness.

*Keep Informed*.   It is essential to have adequate information concerning the medical and psychological aspects of patients' diseases and their personal circumstances. This information provides the appropriate (stimulus) conditions for professionals to understand and at times anticipate patients' behavior. Such conceptualizations minimize the likelihood of being "caught off balance," missing signs that should have been monitored, or even personalizing patients' sometimes demanding and hostile behavior. The latter behaviors, of course, are often patients' responses to their total situation, rather than solely to the caretaker.

*Set Reasonable Expectations for Patients.*   Particularly with severely disabled patients, it is important to set small but attainable goals, rather than large goals or complete recovery as the therapeutic aim. This step-wise, shaping approach stimulates optimal motivation for both patient and staff because it allows frequent, fairly immediate successes while avoiding the frustration and demoralization of failure or of excessively delayed success (see Chapter 3).

*Self-Reward.*   Professionals need to feel comfortable in recognizing their own and others' areas of competence and, when appropriate, in sharing with others good feelings about work. It is important to identify our contributions to patients' improvements and the skillfulness of our efforts despite some patients' limited gains. It is necessary to avoid setting perfectionistic standards of accomplishment or being overly self-critical when uncertain as to the best method of helping a given patient. Rather, it is wise to ask for advice when it is needed and to consider supervision and suggestions from others as an opportunity to learn and improve future performance.

As described for patients in Chapter 3, developing patterns of self-control and self-reward can be quite helpful, and this is applicable to professionals as well as patients. Thus, professionals should plan their schedules to be reinforcing in that they yield a sense of accomplishment and pleasure. Staff members might vary the kinds of patients they care for and plan treatments so that rewarding patients (ones who are improving quickly or who are particularly congenial) follow more difficult ones. We might plan to see a cheerful patient first thing in the morning (to get going) and perhaps just before going home (to leave work feeling good). In addition, plan a few minutes between patients to relax and talk with colleagues, or take a break after finishing several relatively undesirable work chores. Professionals should review their days and consider their patients' improvement. Charting improvement (see Appendix A) often helps the professional as much as the patient to recognize change that may be slow but is substantial when considered within an appropriate time perspective.

*Develop Support among Colleagues.*   Camaraderie among staff often is a key to professionals' emotional survival and commitment to work. The sharing of thoughts, feelings, frustrations, and pleasures encourages intimacies and caring relationships, which provide invaluable support and perspective. Mutual self-disclosure allows coworkers to understand each other and, in turn, respond most helpfully to one another's moods and needs. Healthy families support their members, and work groups must do likewise, especially when members are under conditions of stress. Praise each other's competence, listen when a colleague is having a rough time and needs to talk, and assist when someone needs advice or another pair of hands. Try to avoid petty disagreements or competitiveness and leaving some workers out of the group. Any staff members who are excluded from cliques are likely to become less effective and eventually may leave their jobs. Enjoy praise from one another (rather than deny worthiness), seek help when it is needed, and openly discuss difficulties as they arise. It is a good idea to plan regular meetings for the purpose of reviewing staff morale and discussing interpersonal or work-related issues. Special meetings, perhaps facilitated by a professional consultant, can help to ease particularly difficult situations as they arise, such as the death of a patient who had established close relationships with staff members or the arrival of a child with especially gruesome burns.

*Develop a Balanced Style of Life*.   It is important to seek personal satisfaction (rewards) and revitalization of emotional and physical resources outside of work. We must develop aspects of ourselves other than just our "professional" side. This is particularly true for those engaging in work that is emotionally draining and requires continuous tending to others' needs, as is true of health professionals. It is a mistake to rely solely on work (or any one activity) to provide all of our rewards, such as a sense of accomplishment and self-esteem, intellectual stimulation, and social contacts. Maintaining hobbies, active physical recreation, and friendships beyond the hospital or office will enhance both personal adjustment and capacity for working effectively.

*Learn to Relax*.   Learning to relax can be as important for the professional as for the patient. As mentioned in previous chapters, meditation, yoga, self-hypnosis, or progressive muscle relaxation are several formal methods of relaxation (see Appendix D). Each person also should find relaxing hobbies or diversions, such as gardening, listening to music, walking, taking a sauna, or being massaged. Any form of relaxation can contribute significantly to a sense of well-being and the ability to function optimally.

*Lighten the Workload*.   If symptoms of depression or chronic anxiety persist, it sometimes is necessary to cut down the workload temporarily, for example, by working fewer days per week or less hours per day. Some people find it most helpful to spend the additional free time in recreation, and some prefer to develop other intellectual or professional activities, such as enrollment in classes or professional organizations. Widening interests and sources of satisfaction can moderate depression significantly. For a given stressed individual, lightening his schedule may even involve temporarily or permanently shifting to work with a less chronic or severely ill population. This, however, is relatively rare. In any case, when stress is undiminished after the individual attempts to cope better, it is advisable to seek consultation with work supervisors and perhaps a mental-health professional.

# Epilogue

# The Work of Rehabilitation

## A Case History

In this epilogue we present a case history of one individual's experiences in rehabilitation during the eight months following his injury. The purpose of the case presentation is to illustrate the use of the behavioral techniques that have been described in the foregoing text.

The case history is that of a 31-year-old man who suffered multiple injuries, including a traumatic head injury, in a motor-vehicle accident. Relevant historical information is presented, as well as assessments of functioning in a wide range of skills at various points during the patient's rehabilitation. In accord with this book's focus, we emphasize the patient's emotional, social, and characterological changes and the behavioral strategies used to facilitate his physical recovery and psychological adjustment. We also indicate the importance of cooperation among family members, a multidisciplinary team of rehabilitation professionals, and community agencies.

## Background Information

At the time of his accident, Richard Ellsworth* was a 31-year-old man who had been married for six years and had three children, ages one, three, and four. He was an only child in his family of origin; graduated from high school with Bs and Cs at age 19; served in the military for three years; and then completed community college. He trained to be a long-haul truck driver and proceeded to drive for a living during the next five years. He then worked as a dispatcher for the same trucking firm. He worked the evening shift in this position. Richard's wife, Theresa Ellsworth, was 29 years old, had graduated from high school at 18, worked as a bookkeeper and office manager until her marriage, and then had focused on homemaking and parenting. She was

*Names have been changed to provide anonymity.

considering a return to part-time work. Richard and Theresa had known each
other 18 months before marrying. They grew up in the same suburb of a
medium-sized city and remained in the area after their marriage. The three-
and four-year-old children, both boys, attended preschool five hours a day.
The baby, a girl, stayed home with her mother.

## The Injury

Driving home from work, Richard was struck head-on by a car being driven
the wrong way on the freeway by a driver who was under the influence of
alcohol. Upon admission to the hospital, Richard was in a coma and showed
the following injuries: (1) severe lacerations of the left eye, (2) compound
fracture of the right leg with a shattered right kneecap, (3) internal injuries to
abdomen and liver, and (4) severe head injury with partial right hemiparesis
(right-sided weakness).

## Acute Care

*The Patient.*   Richard's coma lasted for nearly two months, and he received
acute-care hospitalization for two and one-half months. He required a respi-
rator to breathe during his first one and one-half months and was weaned from
the machine gradually during the next month. He underwent multiple
surgeries to remove shattered bones, reset broken bones, repair internal
injuries and hemorrhaging, and repair the corneal lacerations in his left eye. A
CAT brain scan showed mildly dilated ventricles and a low-density area of
lesion in the left frontal region. No neurological surgeries were required.
Richard became increasingly alert and responsive to the environment during
his last three weeks of acute care. He demonstrated mild to moderate agitation, typical for this stage of recovery following traumatic head injury.

## Acute Care

*The Family.*   By Theresa's report, she was advised during the first few weeks
after her husband's injury that he probably would not survive. Expectations
were that, if he did survive, he would have tremendous neurological impairment. Theresa vividly recalled the horror of seeing her husband in emergency, nearly blue and breathing only with the aid of life-support machines. At
one point, after he had been in a coma for weeks, she felt she would have to
decide whether to continue the life supports, but Richard began to breathe
independently. Theresa spent many hours each day at the hospital and had to

assume all responsibilities at home. These functions previously had been divided. Although Richard was well insured, outstanding financial obligations were tremendous. The children required considerable care and were increasingly demanding of attention as familial disruption continued. The youngest child spent weekdays at Theresa's parents' home. When the older children first saw their father as he was nearing the end of acute care, they withdrew from him and denied that this man was, in fact, their father.

## Richard's Inpatient Rehabilitation

Three months of inpatient rehabilitation followed Richard's acute care.

*Medical Status.*   Richard's medical course was relatively smooth after acute care, in that no crises arose. His physical recovery was slow, however, and several areas of marked impairment persisted. A follow-up CAT brain scan showed no sites of lesions and normal ventricular space. His eye and skeletal injuries required continued consultations from ophthalmology and orthopedics. His left eye discriminated light only and was quite disfigured. Prognosis for returned vision was poor, and plastic surgery for cosmetic purposes was advised. The extent of paresis in his right leg initially was unknown, due to the heavy long-leg casting required to reset fractures. In approximately two months, a lighter, short-leg cast allowed evaluation and revealed considerable retained motor function. Bowel and bladder control had been recovered during acute hospitalization, and the one toileting accident, which occurred on the night of Richard's transfer to the rehabilitation ward, appeared to be largely anxiety related. The positioning of his paretic right arm was accomplished with care to avoid undesirable skin pressure and decreased range of motion. His skin was not at high risk to develop ulcers because he changed positions frequently and retained sensation in his paretic side, which allowed pain to cue him to reposition himself. Consultations by a physiatrist (a physician specializing in rehabilitation) continued throughout his hospitalization.

*Neuropsychological Status.*   Upon arrival at the rehabilitation unit, Richard had oriented himself to person and place but not to time. He misreported his own age and the ages of his older children. He knew he had a young infant but could not recall her age or much about her development. He gave a good personal history up to approximately two years prior to injury. More recent memory was spotty, and he had total loss of recall for events occurring between the time of his accident and two to three weeks previous to questioning. He showed confusion and considerable agitation concerning his confinement to the hospital and his sense of lost time. Richard was inadequately aware of his deficits and denied the possibility of permanent physical disability, particularly blindness in his left eye. His speech was fast paced, mildly disinhibited, and disorganized. He showed word-finding problems but could communicate his basic ideas and needs. His behavior was somewhat concrete and his approach to tasks was impulsive, trial-and-error in style, and inadequately monitored. His social style was friendly and disinhibited, and he was quite talkative. He was extremely cooperative with all therapists and consistently optimistic, which was somewhat inappropriate given the seriousness of his condition. Richard also showed emotional lability; he was easily upset and irritated and could not control his emotional expression adequately.

Early in his stay at rehabilitation, Richard was particularly agitated, frequently demanded the nurses' attention (sometimes by screaming from his room), and tried to get up and walk, despite his inability to do so with safety. Without physical restraints he was at risk for a fall, with possible further injury. His being restrained, however, precipitated marked anger and agitation. During the first several nights in the new setting, he reported frightening nightmares. He was most calm and oriented when Theresa was with him.

Initial formal evaluation of cognitive skills revealed diffuse impairment affecting intellectual, characterological, and self-regulatory skills (see Chapter 9). Richard's language skills, although obviously impaired from their projected premorbid level, were relatively intact. He showed good retention of previously learned information (remote memory), knowledge of practical social rules, vocabulary, mental arithmetic, and verbal reasoning. However, he experienced word-finding problems and difficulty with organization of language. His reading, spelling, and arithmetic were significantly below his premorbid levels of achievement. In mathematics, he had forgotten basic operations and made errors due to impulsivity and spatial confusion, as in carrying numbers. His reading deficit suggested poor visual scanning, impulsiveness, and compromised ability in phonetics.

Richard's visual-spatial skills were more significantly compromised than were his verbal skills. He showed a mild left-sided neglect. His motor coordination and motor planning were poor, even considering that he had to use his left hand. He had particular difficulty in recognizing and organizing part-whole relationships, abstract visual-spatial material, and sequences of events shown in pictorial form. These problems impaired, for example, Richard's ability to construct or follow diagrams (mechanical drawings, maps), put puzzles together, and conceptualize sequences and sense in nonverbal, social behavior.

In regard to memory, he showed relatively intact remote recall but significantly impaired short-term memory and new learning. His verbal memory loss appeared further impaired due to his word-finding problem. His retrieval of verbal information was more impaired than was his initial registration of the material. His recall of visual-spatial material was difficult to assess due to his impaired graphic ability with his left hand, but it appeared deficient to at least some extent.

The functional (psychological) components of Richard's adjustment were not discriminated easily from characterological changes secondary to his organic deficits (see Chapter 9). However, his agitation and denial of potential residual impairments were judged to be functional, at least in part. His premorbid style of coping, according to Theresa's reports, seemed consistent with his current style of denial and, at times, naive optimism. His premorbid style also was described as somewhat impulsive, self-conscious, and probably overly eager to please and gain approval.

In terms of treatment strategies, all therapists intially focused on orienting Richard to the rehabilitation setting, moderating his agitation, and gradually helping him to identify deficits so that he could engage most productively in therapies. First, all staff recognized that Richard's agitation was associated with his level of consciousness and was a result of his move to a new, unfamiliar setting. Theresa was asked to be available during the transition, to ease Richard's confusion and anxiety. For the most part, however, nurses were left to manage his agitation and to shape his adjustment to the rehabilitation unit. He was placed in a room close to the nursing station where he could see and hear that others were nearby. Before he mastered use of the call system, staff members responded promptly to his call light and his screams. As each nurse responded, she demonstrated use of the call light, guided Richard's performance, and then attended to his expressed need. Especially because he clearly stated his fear of being alone, nurses visited him frequently, even when he was not soliciting company, and they arranged for him to be out of his room and with others as much as possible. Nurses tried never to criticize him for his agitation and desire for company. Instead, they tried to meet his needs and praise his increasing calm, his tolerance for being alone, and his appropriate manner of seeking reassurance and social support.

To enhance Richard's orientation, information was posted in his room, including basic biographical data such as his age, occupation, family members' names and ages, and the nature of his condition. The current date, names of primary caretakers and therapists, and his daily schedule of activities also were posted. His daily schedule was consistent, and he usually was treated by the same nurses and therapists, in order to provide predictable structure. He was given a book to keep with him at all times to record essential personal data and information regarding daily activities. This diary provided an aid for Richard's impaired short-term memory and a record of behavior for others' reference. Initially, only very basic information was recorded. With his improving orientation, however, more complex and potentially distressing data were recorded to prompt his acknowledgment of deficits. Thus, a list of deficits, complemented by a list of strengths, was prepared. This list was reiterated frequently by staff members, to cue Richard's recognition of deficits and to let him know how these deficits would be approached therapeutically. The list of strengths and assets was as follows.

1. Verbal comprehension
2. Verbal reasoning
3. Remote memory (for old history and much previously learned material)
4. Sense of humor and optimism
5. High motivation/cooperation
6. Congenial social style
7. Strong family support

Table 1 shows the list of deficits and its manner of presentation. As shown, impulsivity, impaired memory, and inadequate self-monitoring (checking work and awareness of deficiencies) were addressed by specific treatments that could be used by all staff members, regardless of the content of their work (nursing, physical exercise, social interaction).

To moderate Richard's impulsivity, all staff members insisted that he allow them to complete their statements or questions before he responded. If he interrupted or answered prematurely, they might say something like, "Wait, now. I'm not quite done. Remember you've got to wait, listen, and then organize your answer before responding." Staff members obviously had to say this in a friendly, nonpunitive style and rely upon previously established rapport. They also could refer to Richard's problem list and recall for him that their comment was consistent with the agreed-upon treatment strategies, rather than an on-the-spot reprimand. In some conversations or tasks, Richard was instructed to say aloud, as a cue to himself, "listen, wait, consider how to answer best" and then to count to five in order to assure delay. Within two weeks, he was observed, without prompting, to guide himself to "wait" and to correct himself for "going too fast and not thinking." His impulsivity and associated lack of organization and careless errors decreased gradually over the next several months. His impulsive style continued to be observed occasionally, however, in a range of tasks, particularly when he was aroused emotionally or fatigued.

Richard's poor self-monitoring ability (problem #5 in Table 1) contributed to two problems. First, he did not listen adequately to his own responses, check his work, and make necessary corrections. Second and more generally, he failed to recognize the extent of his deficits and consequently resisted certain precautions (restraints initially needed for safety) and activities (learning to write with his left hand, which he refused because he insisted that he soon would regain skill in his right hand).

**Table 1**

| Problems | What to Do |
| --- | --- |
| 1. Impulsivity | I must stop, think, and organize before responding. If I behave impulsively, others will interrupt me and tell me to "think before acting." |
| 2. Word finding | Attend speech therapy. I must ask for help and explain what I am trying to say. Others will supply words if I ask them. |
| 3. Visual-spatial organization | Others will remind me to "look to the left" until I begin reminding myself. I should "talk to myself" and use my good verbal skills to help organize what I see and how it hangs together. |
| 4. New learning and memory | Use my diary. Ask people to repeat information and record the main points. When my memory fails, I must ask again for correct information. |
| 5. Not entirely aware of deficits | I must check all work. Others will tell me to do so. Others also will point out my deficits and any errors in performance that I may not be aware of. |

Toward the first problem, Richard's poor self-correcting, a strategy much like that for impulsivity was used. Therapists consistently prompted Richard to review his work or what he had said, decide if his behavior was adequate, and, if not, consider how he could make improvements. Corrective feedback was given only after he had attempted to correct his own work. He was praised for all spontaneous attempts to correct himself, for requesting assistance if he recognized "not knowing" how to proceed, and for improving his performance after prompting to do so. Whenever new skills were taught, therapists emphasized the importance of self-monitoring and modeled this behavior with verbal commentary during their own demonstrations.

Toward the second problem, Richard's denial of his deficits, several approaches were planned. The first steps were initial feedback sessions from therapists in each discipline and the formulation of the problem list presented in Table 1. Professionals prefaced their feedback with statements of their awareness that Richard might disagree or fail to recognize the deficits they listed. His acknowledgment of any deficits was praised, and his disagreement was not pursued. Staff members avoided arguments because confronting his denial probably would not be productive and would be likely to increase his anxiety and to result in interpersonal tension between him and his therapists. Rather, professionals' opinions simply were stated, recorded in Richard's diary, and mentioned repeatedly during therapies. Referring to the list served to alleviate his feeling personally confronted by a therapist who might be identifying a problem with no demonstrable support. Over time, with the repetition of information about deficits, his experience of success and limitations in activities, and his monitoring of improvements or lack thereof, Richard developed greater understanding of his disabilities. His acceptance progressed as he gradually recognized deficits ranging from the least to the most threatening. Emotional support and acknowledgment for retained assets seemed to contribute enormously to his ability to realize and accept that some of his skills were impaired. In addition, his realization of deficits appeared to be facilitated by his socializing with other young head-injured patients. He first recognized others' deficits and then their sometimes poor awareness of their own deficiencies. Seeing this process in others helped him to recognize it in himself. The camaraderie with these patients, and his seeing himself as less impaired than some others, contributed to his feelings of self-esteem and his consequent tolerance of increasingly threatening feedback.

As described previously, Richard's memory was enhanced by the consistent use of a diary, to which he could refer to retrieve lost information and be certain of its accuracy. Staff members also tried to give him information when they approached him rather than ask for information and thereby require him to recall facts, which might have increased his anxiety. For example, when visitors came or staff entered his room, they introduced themselves by name and identified their roles or relationship to him. Continuity of daily activities and therapists also helped him to learn through repetition and habit building. Changes in routines were announced in advance and repeated at intervals, to prompt him to be prepared.

The efficacy of the described treatments was enhanced by Theresa, who consistently modeled her behavior after that of the professionals, and by Richard's own positive attitude and commitment to rehabilitation.

In addition to the strategies just described, which were used across disciplines, speech and language therapy provided specific, intensive training in verbal expression, literacy skills (reading, writing, and arithmetic), memory, and behaviors such as concentration, self-monitoring, and impulse control. Richard was scheduled for two half-hour speech-therapy sessions daily. Initial goals were to improve his concentration, orientation, and impulsiveness. He and the speech pathologist focused on reviewing his personal history, recent events, and daily activities (orientation and memory training). They gradually began focusing on specific language skills such as word finding, organizing expressive language, spelling, reading, and doing mathematics. Along with literacy skills, Richard reviewed phonetic rules and arithmetic operations. He practiced by drilling and was given immediate feedback and guidance for improvement.

Psychological counseling began after Richard was oriented to his current situation and familiar with rehabilitation routines. Initial goals were to enhance his awareness and understanding of his deficits and to moderate his anxiety. At this time, the essential ingredients of counseling consisted of giving him information, listening to his concerns, and providing emotional support and practical guidance. As his cognitive skills and emotional control improved, he was helped to identify specific concerns regarding personal, family, and vocational changes. He was guided in increasingly complex problem solving, praised for adjustive efforts, and given concrete feedback on his performances. During the course of discussions, the psychologist prompted and praised him for organizing his ideas, reflecting before responding, and correcting his own errors. At the hospital, the psychologist and Richard met two times weekly for a half-hour session. After home visits were initiated, one of the meetings became a conjoint counseling session with Richard and Theresa (see Therapeutic Home Visits, later).

*Physical Status.*   Initial evaluation found Richard's leg and arm strength significantly impaired, particularly on the right, and his balance poor. Initial goals were to teach him to move about independently by maneuvering his wheelchair and transferring to and from the wheelchair with minimal assistance, and then to do this independently. To approach the long-term goal of independent ambulation, therapists began shaping Richard's sitting balance, righting response to imbalance, tolerance for sitting upright, and standing balance. Gait training proceeded as the return of some right-leg function became apparent and a lighter, short-leg cast was in place. Richard was scheduled for two half-hour sessions of physical therapy daily. Near the end of his second month in rehabilitation, Richard started practicing ambulation with a walker, and by the time of discharge he was walking well with the walker on many surfaces but continued to use the wheelchair for general mobility. He transferred independently most of the time, but occasionally required help standing up from a sitting position. Throughout the course of physical therapy, managing Richard's behavioral deficits (impulsiveness, compromised judgment, and sometimes overly zealous efforts), discussed in the previous section, played a great role in his ability to learn and perform optimally.

*Activities of Daily Living.*   Initial evaluation revealed restricted range of motion in Richard's right arm and mild fine-motor impairment of the left hand. Goals were to facilitate optimal return of strength, range of motion, and motor control of the right arm and to teach him to manage independently, primarily with his left, nondominant hand.

Richard had two half-hour occupational-therapy sessions daily, one of which was in the morning and designed specifically for work on such self-care as dressing and grooming. His relearning independent grooming, dressing, bathing, and the like depended not only upon his ability to coordinate activities one-handedly but also upon his cognitive ability to concentrate, sequence activities, alternate mental sets as needed, and inhibit impulsive behavior. Verbal cueing helped him to organize his behavior, and he was helped to avoid impulsive errors by consistent prompting and feedback to "wait, consider what to do, then, and only then, proceed." Verbal cues and praise for looking to the left also helped him to compensate for his mild left-sided neglect.

*Social Services.*   As soon as Richard had arrived at the rehabilitation center, before he had even left the hospital, a social worker had begun arranging community resources to help him and his family. Funding was sought through Richard's private insurance company, Social Security Disability, and a county agency to aid victims of crimes (Richard was injured by a drunken driver). A referral also was initiated to the Division of Vocational Rehabilitation. Although Richard clearly was not ready to begin vocational planning and training, this early referral brought him to the attention of the agency and allowed his assigned counselor to become familiar with him and his circumstances over a period of time.

Other relevant community agencies and activities were identified for Richard and Theresa which could complement Richard's inpatient program and continue as sources of assistance after discharge. For example, Theresa was told about a local support and guidance group led by psychologists for spouses of brain-injured individuals. She also was given names of individuals who were in circumstances similar to her own, whom she could contact independently. Similarly, Richard was told about a support and activities group for brain-injured adults. Although he chose not to participate in this group, he did arrange to meet individually with several young brain-injured men and found such meetings to be supportive.

*The Family's Role.*   Initially, the goals for Richard's family, most importantly Theresa, were to orient them to the rehabilitation setting, to let them know what they could expect to happen and how they would be asked to participate in Richard's program, and to enhance their own adjustment. Theresa came every day for several hours during the day. In the evening, she came with the children, who now recognized and showed no fear of their father. Theresa was fully informed of Richard's evaluations and scheduled therapies and was invited to attend the latter. Information concerning Richard's premorbid history was solicited to help professionals to assess changes in his functioning and to properly discriminate behaviors associated with injury from those previously characteristic of him.

Staff members worked to establish rapport with Theresa and let her know how competent she was in helping her husband and managing the family on her own. They also acknowledged, however, how stressful life must be for her and emphasized that she must attend to her own needs as well as to those of her husband (see Chapter 13). Theresa began weekly meetings with the psychologist for guidance and support in both of these areas, namely, interacting most therapeutically with Richard, and coping personally with catastrophic life changes.

As both Richard and Theresa adjusted to rehabilitation routines, Theresa was encouraged to take more time away from the hospital to rest and seek enjoyable diversion with friends and in pleasurable activities. She was encouraged to ask for help from family members and friends; for example, she would ask someone to stay with the children one night so that she could go out, or she would arrange for a friend to visit Richard when he wanted company but she needed a rest.

Theresa's participation in Richard's rehabilitation became increasingly active, as therapists advised her about things that she and he should do on their own, and as she was given a helping role during therapy sessions. This allowed her to understand better Richard's strengths and deficits, and it began preparing her to help Richard on her own at home.

## Therapeutic Home Visits: Richard's Beginning Reentry Home

After approximately two months in inpatient rehabilitation, Richard, Theresa, and therapists agreed that passes out of the hospital would be appropriate. The first pass was for one day, but thereafter passes were for the weekend and included an overnight stay. Theresa and Richard were prepared to manage his transfers in and out of their car, his daily medications, and his continuing self-care. Initially, he was required to use his wheelchair only and not to try walking at home. On the first day pass, they chose to have the children elsewhere so that they could be alone and have minimal distractions during this significant transition. On future passes, the children were at home.

After each home pass, therapists inquired of both of them how they managed specific tasks. The therapists also helped problem-solve any difficulties that arose and reviewed the couple's implementation of suggestions from prior weeks. In consultation with the psychologist, Richard and Theresa typically agreed on areas that needed attention. For example, during the first two passes, Richard reportedly was extremely emotional, easily angered by the children, and tearful for hours in anticipation of returning to the hospital.

The psychologist emphasized the normality of this upset as a result of Richard's long hospitalization, his longing to be well and able to remain at home, and his emotional lability secondary to injury. Richard was helped to identify situations and thoughts that precipitated his emotionality, as well as responses from his wife that perhaps reinforced the undesirable behavior. He then was helped to consider ways to distract himself from negative ruminations that upset him, for example, by listening to music, telling himself that he would be home again shortly, and inviting neighbors over in whose presence he seemed to maintain greater emotional control. Richard decided to arrange some pleasurable activities at the hospital to follow immediately his return at the end of the weekend. This was expected to offer some pleasure (reward) during a particularly depressing period of time. Richard and Theresa also agreed on a way for her to respond to his excessive upsets at home. Although she expressed understanding of his emotionality, they decided it would be best for her to leave him alone when he was excessively upset, rather than risk exacerbating the situation by the reinforcement of sympathy and attention. She agreed, however, to be immediately attentive to him and spend time with him when he maintained his composure or regained control. If he had a specific concern, however, that could be solved by discussion with her, she would use her discretion and listen. These methods worked well; Richard showed markedly decreased tearfulness the following weekend and none thereafter. Of course, his acclimatization over time undoubtedly contributed to his becoming accustomed to the alternation between home and hospital.

Another problem at home was Richard's desire for Theresa's undivided attention and his expectation of help immediately following all requests. He even woke her repeatedly at night to ask for help with things he could manage independently. Theresa felt she was functioning too much as her husband's caretaker and saw herself behaving angrily and with resentment. Both agreed that changes had to be made. For example, they would make sure that Richard's likely needs (urinal, glass of water, remote control for the T.V., telephone) were available to him and within easy reach. If he wanted anything aside from an emergency item, he agreed that he would accept his wife's response that she would get it for him in a little while. She agreed to ask intermittently if he wanted anything and to be sure to sit down and talk with him often when he was not asking for help. Richard also recognized that boredom occasioned quite a bit of his demanding behavior and that his involvement in activities, (helping with household chores, telephoning a friend, reading to the children, practicing writing) could moderate the boredom. Because he still found it difficult to come up with ideas for activities, he and the psychologist drew up a list of possibilities from which he could choose. Certain independent activities such as cooking a meal and doing the laundry were scheduled routinely for different days. Not only did these activities provide Richard with diversion and practice for independent functioning, but they offered a source of reward associated with his mastery of skills, knowledge that he was contributing to the household, and his receiving compliments from his wife for his assistance.

As weekend passes continued, Richard and Theresa attempted increasingly to approach a normal range of activities, including inviting relatives to visit, having friends over, going to a friend's home as a family, and Richard's staying at home alone for increasingly long periods. Reinitiating activities with the children and assuming a parenting role also were important. Richard noted that a firm tone of voice, clear directives, and backup from Theresa allowed his resumption of authority with the children, despite his not being able to run after them or physically coerce compliance if they refused to obey.

The couple's resumption of sexual relations also was discussed prior to home visits. Fortunately, Richard's sexual functioning was not impaired and neither partner found his injuries so distasteful as to forestall sexual activity. Feelings and pragmatic issues, such as positioning of a heavy leg cast and Richard's movement without much voluntary control of his right side, were discussed candidly and suggestions were offered.

As Richard's presence at home became more regular, and especially as his discharge became imminent, Theresa, in her husband's presence, was encouraged to plan weekends to yield her own personal pleasure as well as to assure his satisfaction. The family was to cater less to him, and he was encouraged to focus more on others and less on himself and his accident. This refocusing of conversation and attention was facilitated by practice in communication skills. He was helped to show greater interest in his wife by asking her questions, praising her efforts, and refraining from repetitive descriptions of his own condition. He was prompted to talk about events other than his accident, such as world events, books, or television shows.

## Richard's Outpatient Rehabilitation

After three months of inpatient rehabilitation (thus, five and one-half months subsequent to his injury), Richard was discharged home and scheduled to continue treatment as an outpatient. At discharge, he was independent in a wheelchair, walked with a walker for limited distances with supervision, and transferred independently but, for safety, still with supervision. He was independent in daily self-care, although he required necessities to be set up for him and needed some assistance and equipment (bath bench) in the shower. Richard was able to help in the kitchen, do laundry, vacuum from his wheelchair, and do light dusting, all with the purpose of contributing to household management.

Reassessment of psychological functioning revealed a pattern of skills similar to that on admission but with significant improvements in nearly all areas. Orientation, concentration, recent memory, word finding, and arithmetic skills were improved most notably, although still somewhat deficient. Organization of visual-spatial information remained more significantly impaired. Impulsivity and poor self-monitoring were much improved and interfered less with performance of varied skills. Richard was able to identify his deficits but remained intermittently unrealistic about full recovery and return to his premorbid activities and position of employment. He showed increasing awareness of "personality changes" and expressed feelings of alienation from his past, and in particular, the concern that Theresa might not want to remain married to this "new" person. He said he could understand her potential dilemma but became anxious at the prospect of the marriage breaking up.

Richard was scheduled for therapies at the rehabilitation center four days a week. On each occasion, he had two half-hour sessions of physical therapy, a one-hour session of speech therapy, and a one-hour session of occupational therapy. Once a week, he met with a psychologist for half an hour. Theresa met with the psychologist as well, once a week for one hour.

Richard did not require hourly structure beyond therapy times, but a range of activities was suggested and he kept a log of the new behaviors he performed daily. These steps were reviewed weekly with the aim of broadening his range of activities and independent interests. To facilitate reentry into the community, special weekend activities also were prompted. During his first two months at home, Richard went to a restaurant with the family, went to drive-in movies with Theresa, stayed home with a friend and the children, went to a shopping center, and bought something in a store for the first time in seven months. Each successful venture was savored by him and was supported enthusiastically by Theresa and the therapists. Richard felt decreasingly self-conscious as he received largely positive feedback for the adequacy of his behavior in public. As he became increasingly able to deal with a greater number of situations, Theresa perceived him as increasingly competent. With this, she was encouraged to moderate her role as therapist, and interact with her husband in a more egalitarian manner.

After approximately six weeks, Richard's speech therapy was discontinued because his language functioning was recovered sufficiently to merit this. Further gains were expected to come slowly and as a result of naturally occurring experiences outside of therapy. Physical therapy continued. After two months, he still used a wheelchair for long distances but could walk independently with a cane on smooth surfaces. Independent ambulation was targeted as a goal toward which to work during the next several months. Richard's functioning also was recovered sufficiently, after two months, for occupational therapy to begin focusing less on daily self-maintenance and more on vocational retraining. His previous employer felt that a job could be found for him at the company; therefore, Richard's counselor from the Vocational Rehabilitation Department and his therapist in the rehabilitation center's prevocational program both met with the employer and drew up a list of specific skills Richard would need in order to manage each of several possible jobs. Training him in these specific skills was initiated at the hospital.

Theresa was encouraged to think about both personal and couple-oriented goals that she had left unfinished eight months ago. She was prompted to look for part-time employment in a few months, as she had planned to do prior to Richard's accident. She also was helped to express her fears for the future and assert her right to have mixed emotions about continuing to live with Richard. They both acknowledged that the marriage should not continue *because* of the accident but, rather, could survive happily only if each partner felt that he or she had a choice. Theresa also was helped to structure her participation in a range of new activities that did not focus on Richard. She decided to take both a night-school class in business and a ceramics class, and to continue a monthly card-game meeting and regular nights out with friends.

## Current Status

At the time of this writing, eight months after Richard's injury, physical therapy, vocational training, and psychological counseling continue and probably will for many additional months. Medical, ophthalmological and orthopedic follow-up also continue; and cosmetic surgery for Richard's left eye will be scheduled. The Department of Vocational Rehabilitation will remain involved until Richard returns to some level of employment. Funding from Social Security Disability, the Victims of Crimes program, and insurance agencies also will continue until the family's independent income is reestablished and rehabilitation costs are paid.

# Appendixes

Appendixes

# Appendix A
## *Charting Progress*

The areas of progress to be charted, of course, depend on the patient's particular rehabilitation goals. For example, the number of words spoken each hour may be counted for an aphasic patient, the number of hours tolerated out of bed each day may be tallied for an easily fatigued patient, or all incidents in which conversation is initiated may be recorded for a socially withdrawn patient. Charting often functions as a means of reward because the patient sees a record of accomplishments that otherwise might seem too insignificant to notice. Charts also provide excellent information from which both patient and caretakers can assess the patient's progress and the effectiveness of treatments.

The following are two examples of charting progress with patients. The

Figure 3. The Number of Feet Walked by a Patient during Successive Therapy Sessions.

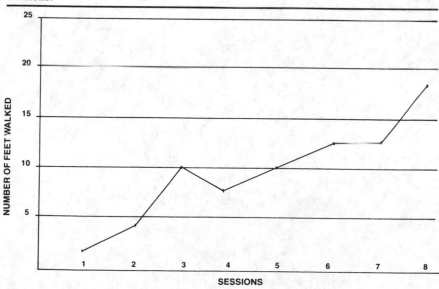

first example (Figure 3) is a line graph that shows the distance walked during successive therapy sessions by a patient who was relearning to ambulate. The second example (Table 2) is a checklist that records attendance in therapy for a patient who was missing scheduled treatments and having difficulty recognizing any rehabilitation successes. Getting to therapy certainly was something this patient could do and, of course, was an obvious precondition for progress in treatment.

Table 2.   A Recording of Therapies Attended by a Patient.

|  |  | Monday | Tuesday | Wednesday | Thursday | Friday |
|---|---|---|---|---|---|---|
| Physical therapy | 9:00– 9:30 | X |  | X | X | X |
| Occupational therapy | 10:00–11:00 |  |  |  |  | X |
| Swimming | 11:00–11:30 | X |  | X | X | X |
| Physical therapy | 1:30– 2:00 |  |  |  | X | X |
| Biofeedback | 2:30– 3:00 |  |  |  |  | X |
| Speech therapy | 4:30– 5:00 |  |  |  |  |  |
| | TOTAL | 2 | 0 | 2 | 3 | 5 |

# Appendix B

## *Examples of Reward and Praise*

A reinforcer or reward is anything a person likes to have or enjoys doing. The following are some ideas of potential rewards for patients.

Visiting with another person
Writing to a friend
Talking on the telephone
A massage
Being outdoors
Reading or being read to
Recording improvement in some
   skill
A hug
Listening to music
A smile and greeting
Cigarettes and an opportunity
   to smoke
Alcoholic drinks
Watching television
Having privacy

Playing cards
Hunting
Wearing makeup
Fragrances
Checking accomplishments off a list
   of "jobs to be done"
Coffee
A "gift"
Money and an opportunity to buy
   things
Fishing
Being at home
Having hair brushed and
   styled
Getting mail
Giving advice

Points or tokens also can become reinforcers for the behaviors they follow if they are exchangeable for already rewarding experiences such as those just listed. For example, each point earned during therapy (for specified behavior) may be exchangeable for a cigarette or some minutes of rest in bed. Or, the accumulation of five tokens may afford a patient an extended visit with a friend or a choice of recreational activities in the evening. The concepts and procedures involved in using token systems are discussed thoroughly in T. Ayllon and N. Azrin's *The Token Economy: A Motivational System for Therapy and Rehabilitation* (1968). Such a system, if used at all in rehabilitation, is seen most often with children or severely impaired patients.

Receiving positive feedback and praise about oneself or one's accomplishments also is rewarding and typically controls a wide range of behavior.

Because it is desirable for patients to be responsive to such social rewards (in part because they are so readily available), praise should be given consistently, even when the patient initially requires more concrete (tangible) rewards (tokens, points, a treat). In time, we would expect praise alone to become sufficiently reinforcing to maintain the patient's appropriate behaviors and thus supplant the need for concrete rewards. Although most expressions of praise and approval are reinforcing, comments that specify what the person is being praised for are particularly helpful. Such "labeled" praise informs the person exactly what she did that was desirable; thus, it increases the likelihood that she will repeat that particular behavior or one closely related to it. The following are examples of praise that may be particularly useful during rehabilitation.

"Great! You're following my instructions exactly."

"Hey, you remembered your schedule. Good memory."

"What a lovely dress. It looks like you've taken a lot of care in grooming today."

"You said the word 'drink' real clearly. Terrific! That's a new word for you."

"I really appreciate your cooperation."

"Even though you weren't sure you'd succeed, you tried. I admire your drive and hard work."

"Good sitting balance . . . muscle control . . . head movement."

"You managed that by yourself. You really are showing more independence. Great."

"I like your initiative in doing exercises on your own. That will help you progress."

A cautionary note: when determining the style and content of compliments, caretakers need to take into consideration the kind of patient with whom they are working. For example, overenthusiastic praise may please one person but alienate another. Subtle and indirect praise, on the other hand, may feel good to some but be missed entirely by others. In general, then, it is important to consider the person's age, cognitive ability, social style, and mood when offering praise and rewards.

# Appendix C

## *Scheduling a Routine*

Daily routines typically should be scheduled in half-hour or one-hour intervals. First, assign times to the most basic activities, such as waking up, going to bed, and eating breakfast, lunch, and dinner. Second, assign times for therapies that may take place at home, a clinic, or a rehabilitation center. Therapies are given priority because of their importance and because therapists may have limited times available. Next, allot time for such self-care routines as washing, bathing, and dressing. These activities should be scheduled in a manner that approximates the patient's past habits, such as dressing before or after breakfast or bathing upon waking or before retiring. Next, allow times for work, exercise, and recreation according to the patient's needs and interests. Allow for rest periods, excursions in the community, and times for socializing. Variety in activities should be planned within the structure of a routine. Special activities, such as seeing a movie or eating out during the week, can offer such variety and serve to lift the patient's spirits. Of course, some flexibility must be maintained to allow for unplanned events, visitors, sickness, and so forth. In addition to scheduling what the patient will do, it is helpful to plan who will be with her or available for assistance if it is needed.

**Table 3. Routine Schedule for Monday.**

| Time | Activity | Who Is Available |
|---|---|---|
| 9:00–10:00 | Get up, drink coffee, wash, and dress | Wife and son are gone; patient's sister comes over to supervise and prepare breakfast |
| 10:00–10:30 | Eat breakfast | Sister |
| 10:30–11:00 | Walk outside | Sister goes home; neighbor is with patient |
| 11:00–11:30 | Garden | Neighbor nearby and watches over fence |

*(continued)*

141

**Table 3.   Routine Schedule for Monday.** *(continued)*

| Time | Activity | Who Is Available |
|------|----------|------------------|
| 11:30–12:30 | Do leatherwork | Home alone with neighbor "on alert" |
| 12:30– 1:00 | Eat lunch | Wife joins patient on her lunch hour from work |
| 1:30– 2:00 | Physical therapy | Wife drives patient to therapy center where he is supervised by therapists |
| 2:00– 2:30 | Socializing in patients' lounge in rehabilitation center | |
| 2:30– 3:30 | Prevocational training | Therapist |
| 3:30– 4:00 | Go home; stop for coffee at restaurant | After school, son picks his father up at the rehabilitation center |
| 4:00– 4:30 | Listen to relaxation tape | Alone in room; son at home |
| 4:30– 5:00 | Play cards or checkers | Son |
| 5:00– 5:30 | Watch TV | Son |
| 5:30– 6:00 | Visit with wife; read paper and discuss events with wife | Wife returns home after work |
| 6:00– 6:30 | Set table for dinner; wash up | Wife and son and occasional visitor in home |
| 6:30– 7:00 | Eat dinner | Son and wife |
| 7:30– 8:30 | Play Scrabble | Son; wife is out with a friend |
| 8:30– 9:00 | Write in diary; call a friend on the telephone | Son |
| 9:00– 9:30 | Bathe and get ready for bed | Wife available for assistance |
| 9:30–10:00 | Get into bed | Wife |

A schedule like this can be made for each day of the week and should be posted in a place that is easily visible to both patient and caretakers. Be sure that the chart itself suits the patient's skills; for example, use large print if the patient has visual problems, use a visually simple design if the patient is distracted easily, or draw pictures if the patient cannot read. It is best to make the schedules in consultation with the patient, since the more he takes part in planning the more likely he is to comply with and enjoy the activities.

# Appendix D

## *Relaxation Training: Imagery*

When a person is under stress or is feeling anxious, he usually has, and may or may not notice, bodily tension. When a person is relaxed or is feeling calm, on the other hand, he usually can notice an absence of significant muscle tension. Therefore, techniques for relaxation have been developed to facilitate the feeling of calmness and relaxation by reducing body tension.

One method of relaxation, called *autogenics*, produces relaxation by the person's evoking images that she experiences as calming. Focusing on these pleasant images mediates the body's relaxation response. This method initially can be accomplished best by somebody, in person, verbally guiding the subject through the images. Later, the subject may choose to practice relaxation on her own and guide herself through the images. Audio tapes on which the relaxation procedures are recorded may be helpful. Such tapes can be requested from rehabilitation therapists or made independently.

The following relaxation procedure takes approximately 20 minutes and should be practiced once or twice daily in a quiet place where there are no distractions, such as television or children who demand attention. The subject should loosen tight clothing, remove glasses or contact lenses, and lie down in a comfortable position with all parts of his body supported by the furniture on which he rests. Lighting should be dim, and the voice of the speaker should be relatively soft and soothing.

The images that are most effective in autogenics are those that reflect the subject's interests and pleasures. It is important to identify the settings, activities, and company that most please the person and to develop procedures based on this information. Details are particularly helpful in stimulating vivid images and usually produce the greatest relaxation response.

The following is an example of an autogenics procedure that was designed for a young man who enjoyed running at the beach, by himself, in sunny, warm weather with a soft breeze blowing.

First, get as comfortable as you can. Lean back. Close your eyes. Allow the bed to support your body so you don't have to exert any physical effort to hold yourself up. Begin tuning out noises and thoughts. Focus all your attention on my voice and on the images you see following my suggestions. Keep your breathing regular. Slow your breathing. Take deep, full breaths. Breathe in, breathe out. Breathe in, breathe out. (Say this in time to the person's breathing.) As you focus on my voice and on your regular breathing, you already may notice yourself feeling more comfortable and relaxed . . . more comfortable . . . more relaxed.

Now, picture yourself in your blue Nikes, your red shorts, and white T-shirt. You're feeling good, and you're ready for a relaxing, long, slow run. The day is beautiful; a blue sky, warm, in the low 80s, and with a cool, lovely breeze. The sand on the beach is warm and clean. The sound of the breeze and of the surf coming to shore is soft, regular, and calming. You are on this beach alone in mid-morning. You begin to run. Long. Slow. Perfectly comfortable with the breeze softly cooling your body and the sound of the surf calming your thoughts. Your breathing stays regular. Breathing in. Breathing out. You move past a favorite tree, a sand castle. . . . Then your thoughts return to yourself, your body, your relaxed sensations. You notice the warmth of your body increasing your state of relaxation. Picture the scene, see yourself running more slowly, more relaxed. Moving down the beach. The sun . . . the breeze . . . the waves . . . the movement . . . your breathing. As you relax, notice the warmth and comfort all over your body . . . your head . . . your jaw . . . your neck . . . shoulders . . . arms . . . off your fingertips. Feel relaxation in your chest . . . your stomach . . . your back . . . thighs . . . down your legs . . . feet . . . off your toes. All over . . . relaxation.

Continue seeing yourself running and allow your comfort to develop further. On your own now, continue feeling the image and furthering your own state of relaxation. (Allow the person two to three minutes to continue the imagery without guidance.)

Good. Now I'll join you again as your run slows down. You are quite relaxed. You stop running, walk a bit, then lie on the sand. Continue breathing regularly. Enjoying the sun . . . the breeze . . . the sound of the surf. As you become ready, you will alert yourself slowly, put your images away for awhile, and come back in thought to the current time and place. At your pace, when you are ready. You can take your state of relaxation with you as you leave your image. You can come back to this room breathing regularly, feeling calm, feeling more relaxed, and enjoying your feelings.

# Appendix E

## *Resources: Information, Support, and Action*

Many of our communities, citizens' groups, and private foundations, as well as the federal and state governments, have become increasingly concerned with helping disabled individuals to live fuller lives. Consequently, there are hosts of resources available to provide assistance for various needs of the disabled. It is important of course, that interested individuals know how to find and utilize the services that are available. The patients who make appropriate use of community facilities are most likely to regain optimal independence and support and adjust satisfactorily to life with some disability. Because a person is more likely to use these facilities if she makes contact while still in a rehabilitation setting, health professionals should familiarize her with available services and help initiate contact with appropriate agencies prior to discharge from hospital or rehabilitation facilities. This appendix will try, in a very general way, to acquaint health providers with the kinds of resources available and the ways to assist patients in securing services within their communities.

### Locating Services and Information

In health-care settings, social workers typically are the professionals most knowledgeable about community resources and particularly about funding for hospital and rehabilitation services and for financial support if the patient is currently not able to earn a living. There are services provided in the patient's home to aid particular kinds of patients (geri-aides for older people, hospice care for the terminally ill) and to provide particular services (nursing, therapy, meal preparation, housekeeping). Full-time residences such as nursing homes and retirement communities also offer a range of assistance and supervision on their premises. Social workers typically explore these community options with the patient and initiate appropriate referrals during the patient's hospitalization. Once a patient is home, however, it remains a good strategy to call the social service department at a local hospital if questions arise regarding community assistance.

Rehabilitation therapists also should be able to inform the patient about resources in their particular disciplines. For example, a psychologist would know about therapy and support groups; a physical therapist would know about swimming, gyms, and other therapeutic options; and so on. Thus, patients and their families should ask for direction from their therapists as well as their social worker.

Patients and their families also can identify resources independently. For example, the telephone book in many cities is organized in a fashion that makes services for the disabled reasonably easy to locate. Government resources are listed under "United States" or under the name of the patient's city of residence, and organizations are identified according to the services offered or the population with which the service is concerned. In many cities, there is a listing for the United States Government Information Center, which can provide information regarding federal, state, or local services appropriate for particular situations.

The local public library is an excellent source of information. The library often has a collection of government pamphlets, books, and periodicals from different associations for the disabled. The librarian should be consulted to help find desired materials. Libraries also offer a number of free services from the Library of Congress Division for the Blind and Physically Handicapped. For example, the Library of Congress provides lists of "talking books" and audio taped recordings of standard periodicals for visually impaired individuals.

## General Resources in Rehabilitation

To acquaint the patient with the large variety of information and services available, it is advisable to start with a general guide to resources for the disabled. One such reference is *The Source Book for the Disabled: An Illustrated Guide to Easier, More Independent Living for Physically Disabled People, Their Families, and Friends*, edited by Glorya Hale (1979). This book discusses a wide range of needs associated with different disabilities and is a veritable gold mine of information. It gives excellent descriptions of problems encountered by disabled persons, as well as the devices and services available for assistance. One section presents an annotated list of books, organizations, and agencies directed toward specific problems and patient populations. Rather than attempt to reorganize the same information here, we refer our readers to this source book.

Another source of extensive information is the National Rehabilitation

Information Center (the Catholic University of America, Washington, D.C. 20064). This agency searches published material and offers a bibliography on any of a wide variety of rehabilitation topics. Thus, any interested party may initiate a search on, for example, brain injuries or the emotional adjustment to cancer, and receive an annotated bibliography along with, in many cases, an option to purchase copies of specific references.

There is a newly created United States Department of Education, within which are the Bureau of Education for the Handicapped, the Rehabilitation Services Administration (RSA), the Office for Handicapped Individuals (OHI), and the Architectural and Transportation Barriers Compliance Board (ATBCB). Each of these agencies could be contacted for information regarding their services and for directions to appropriate agencies when a particular service is being sought.

We also refer health professionals to a journal, *Rehabilitation Psychology* (Springer Publishing Company, 200 Park Avenue South, New York, New York 10003), for articles on research and treatment with different rehabilitation populations. Occasionally, special volumes focus on a particular rehabilitation issue, such as sex and disability (1978, volume 25, #2), spinal-cord injury (1978, volume 25, #1), and professional and client viewpoints in rehabilitation (1973, volume 20, #1). Other journals that focus upon rehabilitation can be found across a wide range of disciplines, such as medicine, nursing, pediatrics, and vocational services.

## Organizations

Many organizations for disabled people publish leaflets and journals that are available at little or no charge. This material can inform the patient about medical, physical, and psychological facets of his disability and about new ideas and equipment that may improve the quality of his life. Many of these organizations also draw their members into relatively active participation in lobbying for better opportunities, helping each other, and generating money for research. Such participation can be a positive force in helping patients look beyond their own immediate problems to develop a sense of meaning and belonging from their activities. The following is a small sample of the organizations available.

The American Coalition of Citizens with Disabilities, Inc.
1346 Connecticut Avenue, N.W., Washington, D.C. 20036.
National Association of the Physically Handicapped
2810 Terrace Road, S.E., Washington, D.C. 20020.
National Rehabilitation Association
1522 "K" Street, N.W., Washington, D.C. 20005

The National Easter Seal Society for Crippled Children and Adults
22023 West Ogden Avenue, Chicago, Illinois 60612
The Council for Exceptional Children
1920 Association Drive, Reston, Virginia 22091

Other organizations are involved with more specific concerns of the disabled, for example, sports, dancing, or communication with other disabled individuals. Some of these organizations are as follows.

American Association for Health, Physical Education, and Recreation Programs for the Handicapped
1201 16th Street, N.W., Washington, D.C. 20036.

Colorado Wheelers (square dancing)
525 Meadowlark Drive, Lakewood, Colorado 80226

People to People, International Headquarters
2201 Grand Avenue, Kansas City, Missouri 64108

Nearly every kind of disabling condition has its own or several organizations dedicated to research and/or service for those affected by the condition. For example, for spinal-cord injuries there is the National Paraplegia Foundation, 333 N. Michigan Avenue, Chicago, Illinois 60601. For ostomy patients there is the United Ostomy Association, 111 Wilshire Boulevard, Los Angeles, California 90017. For epileptic patients there is the Epilepsy Foundation of America, 1828 L Street, N.W., Washington, D.C. 20036. Many of these associations have local chapters in a great number of cities. Support groups, such as Stroke Clubs and One Day At A Time (for people with cancer) frequently are available locally as well. These local groups can be found through national registries, the telephone book, or by asking a professional working in rehabilitation.

## Publications: Pamphlets and Books

As already mentioned, local, state, and federal agencies publish information concerning many medical conditions and their treatments. For example, the American Heart Association publishes *After a Heart Attack* (1979) for cardiac patients; and (1) *Strokes: A Guide for the Family (1969)*, (2) *Aphasia and the Family* (1969), and (3) *Stroke: Why Do They Behave That Way?* (Fowler and Fordyce, 1974) for stroke patients. The Association for Brain Tumor Research publishes a *Primer of Brain Tumors* for patients with cerebral tumors and their families. Caretakers and patients should contact the appropriate agency and request available information.

Books also have been written about most of the common concerns of disabled people, from sex to employment. There are books on how to manage in a wheelchair, plan appropriate clothing, plan your home, improve your sex life, manage parenting, find new career opportunities, and on and on. There also are books directed toward specific forms of disability, for example, amputation, spinal-cord injury, epilepsy, and renal failure. Many of the books are written by professionals who specialize in rehabilitation, and many are written by the disabled people themselves, in the hope that others will benefit from their experiences. Such books can be found in reference lists in volumes such as *The Source Book for the Disabled* (Hale, 1979) and in the subject catalogue at the library. National services such as the Institute for Information Studies and the ERIC Clearinghouse on Handicapped and Gifted Children (part of the Council for Exceptional Children) also offer lists of relevant publications.

As in most areas of investigation and search, talking frequently with professional colleagues and with patients and their families is an excellent way to "get on the grapevine" and to exchange information, references, and ideas.

# References and Suggested Readings

American Heart Association. *After a Heart Attack*. Dallas: American Heart Association, 1979.

American Heart Association. *Aphasia and the Family*. Dallas: American Heart Association, 1969.

American Heart Association. *Strokes: A Guide for the Family*. Dallas: American Heart Association, 1969.

Association for Brain Tumor Research. *A Primer of Brain Tumors*. Chicago: Association for Brain Tumor Research, 1978.

Athelstan, G.; Scarlett, S.; Thury, C.; and Zupan, I. "Psychological, Sexual, Social and Vocational Aspects of Spinal Cord Injury: A Selected Bibliography." *Rehabilitation Psychology*, 25:1, 1978.

Ayllon, T., and Azrin, N. *The Token Economy: A Motivational System for Therapy and Rehabilitation*. New York: Appleton-Century-Crofts, 1968.

Bandura, A. *Principles of Behavior Modification*. New York: Holt, Rinehart and Winston, 1969.

Barker, R.; Wright, B. A.; Meyerson, L.; and Gonick, M. R. *Adjustment to Physical Handicap and Illness: A Survey of the Social Psychology of Physique and Disability*, New York: Social Science Research Council, 1953.

Beck, A. T. *Depression: Clinical, Experimental and Theoretical Aspects*. New York: Harper & Row, 1967.

Becker, W. C. *Parents Are Teachers*. Chicago: Research Press, 1971.

Benson, D. F., and Blumer, D. (eds.). *Progressive Aspects of Neurologic Disease*. New York: Grune & Stratton, 1975.

Bernstein, D., and Borkevec, T. *Progressive Relaxation Training*. Champaign, Ill.: Research Press, 1975.

Buck, W. M. *Dysphasia: Professional Guidance for the Family and Patient*. Englewood Cliffs, N.J.: Prentice-Hall, 1968.

Butler, R. N. *Why Survive? Being Old in America*. New York: Harper & Row, 1975.

Chipouras, S.; Cornelius, D.; Daniels, S. M.; and Makas, E. *Who Cares? A Handbook on Sex Education and Counseling Services for Disabled People*. Washington, D.C.: George Washington University Press, 1979.

Cooper, I. S. *Living with Chronic Neurologic Disease: A Handbook for Patient and Family*. New York: Norton, 1976.

Cullen, J. W.; Fox, B. H.; and Ison, R. N. (eds.). *Cancer: The Behavioral Dimensions*. New York: Raven Press, 1976.

Eisenberg, M. G. "Sex and Disability: A Selected Bibliography." *Rehabilitation Psychology, 25: 2*, 1978.

Ferster, C. B. and Perrott, M. D. *Behavior Principles*. New York: New Century, 1968.

Fordyce, W. F. *Behavioral Methods for Chronic Pain and Illness*. St. Louis: C. V. Mosby, 1976.

Fowler, R. S. and Fordyce, W. F. *Stroke: Why Do They Behave That Way?* Seattle: Washington Heart Association, 1974.

Goldfried, M. R. and Merbaum, M. (eds.). *Behavior Change through Self-Control*. New York: Holt, Rinehart and Winston, 1973.

Goldiamond, I. "A Diary of Self-Modification." *Psychology Today*, November, 1973.

Gordon, T. *Parent Effectiveness Training*. New York: New American Library, 1970.

Griffith, U. E. *A Stroke in the Family: A Manual of Home Therapy*. New York: Delacorte Press, 1970.

Hale, Glorya (ed.). *The Source Book for the Disabled: An Illustrated Guide to Easier, More Independent Living for Physically Disabled People, Their Familes, and Friends*. London: Imprint Books, 1979.

Heilman, K. M., and Valenstein, E. (eds.). *Clinical Neuropsychology*. New York: Oxford University Press, 1979.

Institute for Information Studies. *Rehabilitation Engineering Sourcebook*. Falls Church, Va.: Institute for Information Studies, 1979.

Kastenbaum, R. (ed.). *New Thoughts on Old Age*. New York: Springer, 1969.

Kerr, N. "Understanding the Process of Adjustment to Disability." *Journal of Rehabilitation*, November–December, 1961.

Kübler-Ross, E. *Death: The Final Stage of Growth*. Englewood Cliffs, N.J.: Prentice-Hall, 1975.

Kübler-Ross, E. *On Death and Dying*. New York: Macmillan, 1969.

Leviton, G. "Professional and Client Viewpoints on Rehabilitation Issues." *Rehabilitation Psychology, 20:1*, 1973, 1–80.

Lezak, M. D. *Neuropsychological Assessment*. New York: Oxford University Press, 1976.

Lezak, M. D. "Living with the Characterologically Altered Brain Injured Patient." *Journal of Clinical Psychiatry, 39*, 1978, 592–598.

Lipp, M. R. *Respectful Treatment: The Human Side of Medical Care*. New York: Harper & Row, 1979.

Lofquist, L. H. (ed.). *Psychological Research and Rehabilitation*. Washington, D.C.: American Psychological Association, 1960.

Luria, A. R. *The Working Brain*. New York: Basic Books, 1973.

Meichenbaun, D. *Cognitive-Behavior Modification: An Integrative Approach*. New York: Plenum Press, 1977.

Moos, R. H. (ed.). *Coping with Physical Illness*. New York: Plenum Medical Book Co., 1977.

Moss, C. S. *Recovery with Aphasia: The Aftermath of My Stroke*. Chicago: University
   of Illinois Press, 1972.
Patterson, G. R., and Gullion, M. E. *Living with Children*. Chicago: Research Press,
   1968.
Pincus, J. H., and Tucker, G. J. *Behavioral Neurology*. New York: Oxford University
   Press, 1978.
Roberts, S. L. *Behavioral Concepts and the Critically Ill Patient*. Englewood Cliffs,
   N.J.: Prentice-Hall, 1976.
Seigman, M. *Helplessness: On Depression, Development and Death*. San Francisco:
   W. H. Freeman, 1975.
Selye, H. *The Stress of Life*. New York: McGraw-Hill, 1956.
Selye, H. *Stress without Distress*. New York: New American Library, 1974.
Shontz, F. C. *The Psychological Aspects of Physical Illness and Disability*. New York:
   Macmillan, 1975.
Skinner, B. F. *The Science of Human Behavior*. New York: The Free Press, 1953.
Task Force on Concerns of Physically Disabled Women. *Providing Family Planning
   Services to Physically Disabled Women*. New York: Human Sciences Press, 1978.
The Junior League of Portland, Oregon. *Circling the City*. Portland, Ore.: 1978.
Walsh, K. W. *Neuropsychology: A Clinical Approach*. New York: Churchill Living-
   stone, 1978.

# Index

# Index